TRANSFER FACTOR AGAINST INHUMAN TERRORISTS

The Mission of this Super Supplement is to save humanity from disease.

Clive J. Buchanan
The Lion of the Platform

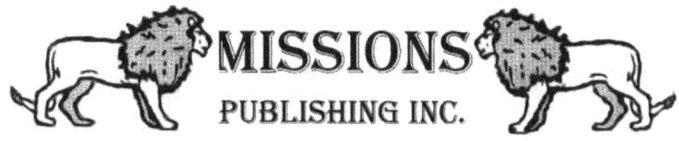

MISSIONS PUBLISHING INC.

Missions Publishing
PO. Box 1537
St. George, UT 84771
Call us toll-free 1-888-344-3892
clive@cjbuchanan.com

The information in this book is for educational purposes only and is not recommended as a means of diagnosing or treating an illness. All matters concerning physical and mental health should be supervised by qualified health practitioners knowledgeable in treating that particular condition. Neither the publisher nor author directly or indirectly dispense medical advice, nor do they prescribe any remedies or assume any responsibility for those who choose to treat themselves.

Printed in the United States of America.

Dedicated to the scientists who devote their lives to finding ways to prolong life and improve the quality of it. It is also dedicated to those who work tirelessly to spread the knowledge of life changing supplements to the world.

Special thanks to Beverly, Sue, Marty, and David who convinced me to investigate the benefits of Transfer Factor and ultimately to write this book.

Thanks to Rita, Constance, Kelly, Norma, Sarah, Laura, Bonnie, Cal, and Bill for their many contributions, suggestions, and corrections.

TABLE OF CONTENTS

CHAPTER 1
PART ONE

THE WAR IS REAL!

THE THREAT IS EMINENT!

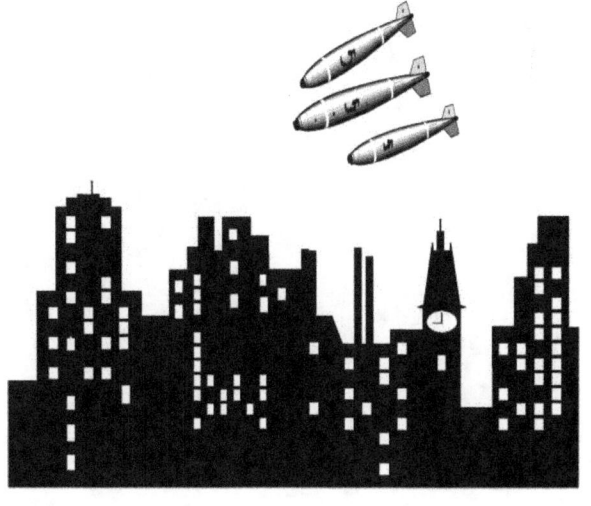

The tips came from a reliable source, the chief surgeon at University of Utah Medical School and the apartment building owner. There are terrorists in the building. They are moving from complex to complex maiming, torturing, and murdering. The wake of destruction is devastating. Some of the tenants are fighting back and dying in the attempt to stop them.

The police have arrived but seem helpless. There are units of the Utah Highway Patrol, Salt Lake Police Department, and the FBI. The Highway Patrol and Salt Lake Police keep sending people into the building. The officers are armed with guns, grenades, mace, and sticks. It sounds unbelievable but they either die or come out empty. The enemy seems to elude them.

> The CIA, NSA, and Home Land Security with all their intelligence gathering sources are of little help. These terrorists strike without warning.

The FBI is firing canister after canister of tear gas into the building but the terrorists seem immune. The only damage being done is to the building and its legitimate tenants. This group of terrorists has developed protective shielding and cloaking devices that protect them from all the weapons of the FBI. It appears as if the building will soon collapse. As the tenants abandon the doomed location the police stand helplessly by as the terrorists escape disguised as tenants. Still others boldly show their true faces having developed protective means of evading the FBI's most powerful weapons. As the FBI fires fragmentation shells from its 155 howitzers, large portions of the building are destroyed. Occasionally, a terrorist falls yet about 50% of the known terrorists escape.

Among the chaos, reports continue to come in of innocent victims being maimed or killed by friendly fire. The police say the terrorists are creating circumstances that make it appear that civilians are enemy targets.

If you were to read this report in the morning paper, on the web, or heard it on the radio or TV you would be both shocked and horrified. Daily fear could become a part of your life. Yet, **the report is true.** It is going on every day in every city, town, and village in the world.

The Inhuman Terrorists are not bomb throwing extremists. They are viruses, bacteria, fungi, yeast, mold, and parasites. The apartment buildings are the bodies of all organic life. You and I own a building that is constantly under attack.

The City and State police are our bodies' immune system. The FBI represents all those who give us medical care. The guns, grenades, mace, and nightsticks are our defence mechanisms. The gas canisters, howitzers, bombs and other weapons of destruction are the tools of our caregivers.

We are engaged in a new kind of war against a largely unseen enemy. Many of the enemy have not yet been isolated or identified. Others have adapted and become immune or resistant to our formidable array of herbs and drugs. AIDS, Tuberculosis, E. Coli, Cancer, Pneumonia, and Gonorrhea are examples of conditions that are either resistant or immune to most or all medications. Some diseases like Tuberculosis were thought to be all but eliminated. Today, Tuberculosis is found in virtually all major cities in the world. Gonorrhea was once cured with a simple shot of penicillin but today it is hard to kill.

Are we doomed to lose this war? Will our generation see the end of mankind? No! Thanks to a relatively unknown hero we will win this war. This hero has only recently become available, in quantity, to the general public. The hero's name is "Transfer Factor".

Chapter 2
Who and What is Transfer Factor?

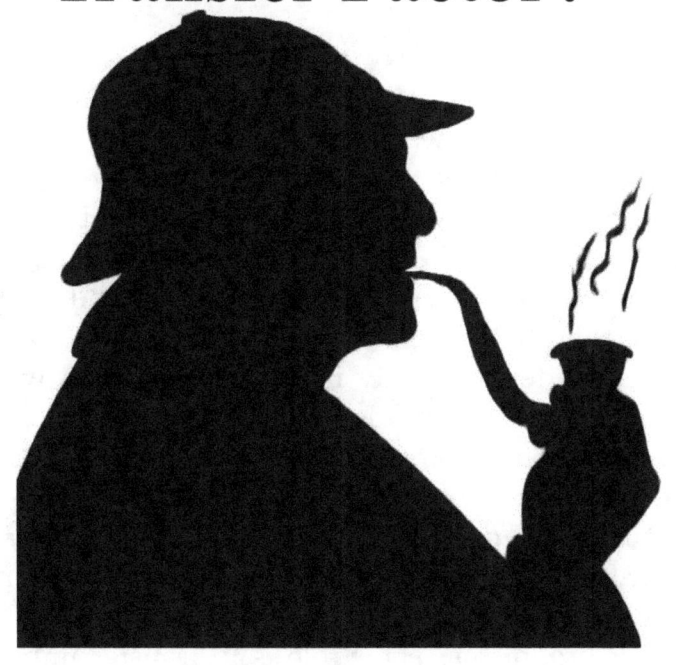

Is this super hero a miniature version of Superman who flies through the body fighting germs and parasites? No! Transfer Factor is an educator that teaches our immune system to discern who and what to attack. It works like a cross between a college professor and a pep squad educating and encouraging greater effort from our white blood cells and other body defense systems. There are many different transfer factors. In this book these factors, as a group, will be called Transfer Factor.

In the first chapter we painted a picture of police fighting a hopeless battle against terrorists. The local police had all the weapons necessary to win the war but they could not see or recognize the enemy. This goes on every day in our bodies. Harmful viruses, parasites, fungi, mold, and bacteria disguise themselves as benign residents of the body. The human body is well armed and ready to handle most invaders but only if it can distinguish which invaders are harmful and which are friendly. Transfer Factor helps the body know the good from the bad. Dr. William J. Hennen, Ph.D. in his book *Natural Immune Booster Transfer Factor* explains Transfer Factor this way, "Transfer Factors are small immune messenger molecules that are produced by higher organisms. Their role is to transfer immune recognition signals between immune cells and thereby assist in educating naïve immune cells about a present or potential danger."

Transfer Factor holds the secrets, intelligence, and knowledge to break the codes of the inhuman terrorists who invade our bodies. This makes it possible to destroy and eliminate enemy cells. Transfer Factor communicates these secret codes and teaches the Good Cells (Our allies), which cells are terrorists. It gives detailed instructions on how to attack and kill them. It reveals their weaknesses.

There is an old joke about the common cold. "If you get a cold and see a doctor right away you will only have to suffer for about a week, but if you don't see the doctor, you will suffer seven long days." The reason the joke is funny is because it is true. When you are exposed to a cold virus it can take as long as five days before the body knows what it is fighting.

Once the specific cold virus is recognized and identified the body's antibodies and NK cells make short work of the virus. The dreaded cold that normally lasts seven days (168 hrs) is usually eliminated within 24 to 72 hours (1-3 days) after it is recognized and identified. If the virus is recognized as a villain when it first enters the body, it is often eliminated before there is the first symptom of the disease.

A little history

Our super hero, Transfer Factor was first discovered way back in 1949. Since then, millions of dollars have been spent researching it. Countless hours have been exhausted trying to isolate it in a cost effective manner.

Dr. H. Sherwood Lawrence discovered Transfer Factor while studying tuberculosis. He took an extract of white blood cells from a person who had fully recovered from tuberculosis and injected it into a patient who had recently contracted the disease. The patient recovered remarkably fast. He concluded that an immune response could be transferred from one person to another. His studies showed that the extract from the white blood cells contained a factor or molecule that transferred immunity. He named this immunity sharing substance "Transfer Factor".

Why was the uncovering of Transfer Factor not heralded as the greatest discovery of all time? Because it came at a time when many new antibiotics were being discovered. History may well call this time the beginning of the antibiotic age. Researchers of the time believed that by the turn of the century all infectious disease would be wiped out.

Between 1949 and 1985 scientists and futurists seemed to fall into one of two camps. One group thought World War III and nuclear winter would kill us all. The other expected Utopia by the year 2000. Students in the sixties and seventies were told that our biggest problem in the year 2000 and beyond would be deciding what to do with our spare time. All of our problems would be solved. In 1970 the Surgeon General of the United States seemed convinced of a rosy future when he declared, "The war against infectious diseases has been won!" In the immortal words of my seven-year old, "Boy was he wrong!"

If foresight were as good as hindsight, there would be no point in living. We would know everything that would happen and life would be dull and monotonous. Real life is full of unexpected surprises. Most of us frequently wake up and find we are walking in the wrong direction from time to time. It is part of what makes life fun and interesting.

$$\left(\begin{array}{c} \textbf{Unexpected surprises} \\ \textbf{are part of what makes} \\ \textbf{life fun and interesting} \end{array} \right)$$

Doctors are mortal too. They, like the rest of us, go in wrong directions from time to time. There was a time when they were into bloodletting. Using leaches was a common practice. Then there was the mercury period when some practitioners gave patients mercury for almost everything. More recent was the cholesterol phobia. People took all cholesterol out of their diet only to discover that eating absolutely no cholesterol raises cholesterol in the blood stream. Conventional bias caused prejudice against such a simple solution as Transfer Factor. They could not believe that Transfer Factor was the answer to most, if not all, our immunological problems. You know the old saying, "If it sounds too good to be true…"

Finding and isolating Transfer Factors was a more complex challenge than finding and isolating a single chemical like those found in most standard pharmaceutical drugs. For these and many other reasons the quest to find commercially practical applications was pushed to a back burner by most researchers. The good news is that the research never stopped. China, Italy, Poland, Romania, and a few American scientists nobly continued the work. It was used on a limited number of patients for an equally limited number of conditions. The technology to make it commercially practical did not exist. In fact, there were no sure fire ways to be sure that the Transfer Factors isolated were potent and viable.

Real progress began when doctors G. B. Wilson and H. H. Fudenberg discovered a method of effectively evaluating and testing Transfer Factor extracts. In 1983 they were issued US Patent No. 4,610,878. The name of the Patent like the process is very complex, "Use of in vitro Assay Techniques To Measure Parameters Related To Clinical Applications of Transfer Factor Therapy". This discovery set the stage for the next advancement.

In November of 1984 Doctors Gregory B. Wilson and Gary V. Paddock applied for a patent on extracting Transfer Factor from colostrum or milk. They received their patent in March of 1989. The process continues to be improved and new patents are being applied for. Today Transfer Factor can also be extracted from the yolk of an egg

Since Transfer Factor's discovery in 1949 an estimated $40,000,000 has been spent on research. In excess of 3,000 scientific papers extolling the virtues or vices of Transfer Factor have been published. Before Doctors Wilson, Paddock, and Fudenberg made their breakthrough discoveries some studies were negative while others were positive. Today virtually all studies are turning out positive. There have been no negative side effects reported from Transfer Factor extracted from pure colostrum or egg yolks.

On January 20, 1998 a major effort to market Transfer Factor was launched by David and Bianca Lisonbee. They and their associates are rapidly making Transfer Factor a household word. Their company is the only U.S. company selling Transfer Factor harvested using the colostrum extraction method patented by Wilson and Paddock at this time. This method is considered by many to deliver the broadest spectrum of viable transfer factors.

If you are the type person who enjoys reading scientific papers Dr. William J. Hennen, Ph.D. lists over 200 of the best Transfer Factor articles in his two books, *Natural Immune Booster Transfer Factor* and *Enhanced Transfer Factor*. Both books are information packed and should be on your must read list if you really want to understand Transfer Factor.

Chapter 3
How Real Is the Risk?

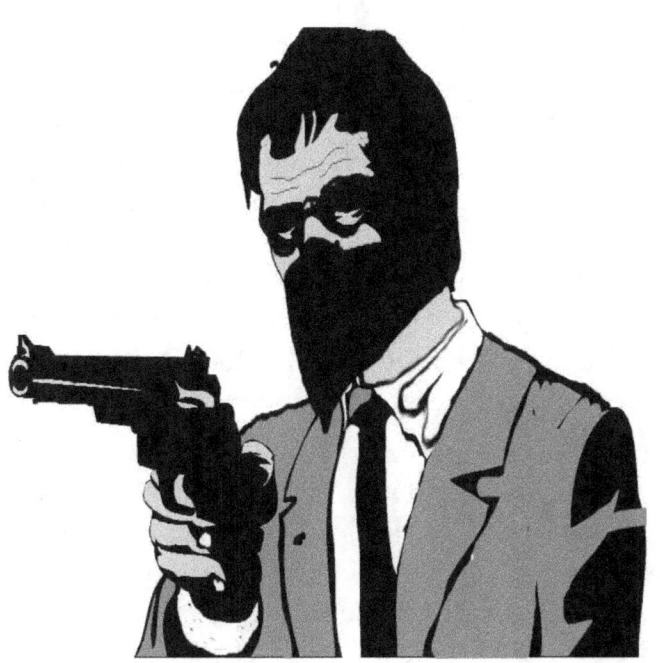

When terrorists mailed anthrax to prominent government officials and members of the press, there was a worldwide panic. Many people started taking anti anthrax medicine in spite of its possible side effects. Yet in the state of New York more people died of the flu between September 11 and January than died of anthrax. The flu is only one of hundreds of diseases killing our people. These Inhuman Terrorists are very active.

We may think we live in a sanitary environment. It is certainly more sanitary than the world experienced a hundred years ago. However, our world is still a dirty place. We have no qualms about setting an apple on our desk and nibbling on it as we get hungry. A recent study by the University of Arizona may change your mind. They found, on average, that 10 million bacteria can be found at any given office desk, phone, and keyboard. To put this in perspective the number of bacteria in your workspace exceeds the number found on the average toilet seat by 400 times. These terrorists are everywhere.

Scientists around the world spend millions of dollars every year trying to invent new strains of deadly bacteria and viruses in the name of self-defence. They call it bacterial warfare. Some third world countries do it because they want to bring the rest of the world to their level or below. Developed countries do it so they can do it back to anyone who does it to them. No matter what the reason, it really is not sound thinking.

Is bacterial warfare a real risk? Every American soldier is trained to survive it. To date there has never been a weapon that has not been used. Before World War II nobody believed that anyone would ever drop an atomic bomb, but the United States did. In the Gulf war there is evidence that the Iraqis used biological weapons.

Sometimes we have the illusion that we are safe, but the Inhuman Terrorists are around us everywhere. We don't know when or how we will be attacked. Every now and then we hear about some poor victim who has contracted a flesh eating disease. I have a cousin who had the bad luck to be bitten by a wood tick. She developed Lyme disease. There are those who believe cancer is caused by either parasites or viruses. Chronic Fatigue Syndrome and Epstein-Barr virus are now common every day words. Doctor Hennen in his book *Transfer Factor* lists a full page of diseases that have become resistant or immune to antibiotics.

Chapter 4
Inhuman Terrorists Disguised as Chronic Disease

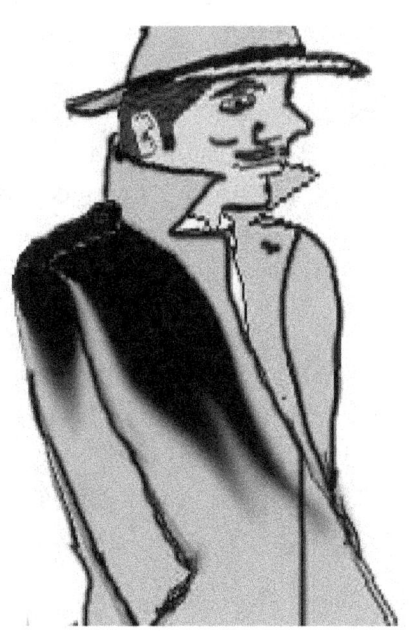

Paul Ewald, a biology professor at Amherst College and author of the book *Evolution of Infectious Disease,* and Gregory M. Cochran, a physicist, have advanced the theory that chronic disease is, in most cases, really infectious disease. They suggest that if Darwin's law of evolutionary fitness and natural selection is valid, then negative traits would be eliminated. Inherited disease that would interfere with reproduction and survival would be quickly eliminated.

If Darwin was right, common illnesses like Alzheimer's, cancers, diabetes, heart disease, and obesity would be eliminated. They could not be genetic diseases. If they are not genetic diseases then they must be infectious diseases or caused by environmental conditions. Ewald and Cochran hypothesize these conditions are caused by inhuman terrorists, namely bacteria, viruses, fungus, mold, and parasites.

Ewald and Cochran are no longer alone. A growing number of scientists believe that inhuman terrorists are actually causing many chronic diseases, long thought to be caused by environment, genetics, and lifestyle. Bacteria, fungus, mold, parasites, and viruses are being exposed as the real culprits.

Just a few years ago the world believed that stomach ulcers were caused by stress and/or stress combined with heredity. The most common treatment was bland food and antacids. Tagamet and Zantac were two of the drugs of choice. The symptoms were often temporarily relieved but the problem remained. The drugs have their own set of possible side effects. These include: bruising, confusion, constipation, diarrhea, dizziness, diminished sex drive, fever, fatigue, hair loss, headache, hives, irregular heartbeat, muscle cramps or pain, rash, slow or fast heartbeat, sore throat, unusual bleeding, and weakness.

A few nutritional enthusiasts got rid of their ulcers using Cabbage Juice, Capsicum, or Propolis. They did not know why it worked. They just knew it did work. They were killing terrorists and didn't know it.

Today the lion's share of evidence suggests that a bacterium called *Helicobacter pylori (H. pylori.)* is the real villain and cause of ulcers.

Is cancer a front for a Terrorist organization? Is it possible that all cancer is caused by Inhuman Terrorists? We know that human papilloma virus, hepatitis B virus, Epstein-Barr virus, human T-cell lymphotropic virus, and Kaposi's sarcoma-associated herpes virus all cause cancer. Scientists have found conclusive proof. They account for 10 to 20% of cancer cases worldwide.

Cervical cancer is the fifth most common cancer in humans and the second most common cause of cancer death in women. Human papilloma virus (HPV), a sexually transmitted disease, causes most cervical cancer.

Could it be that parasites, fungus, mold and bacteria also play a role?

Hulda Regeher Clark, Ph.D., N.D. in her book *The Cure for all Cancers* claims that parasites play a role in all cancers. She further claims that if you get rid of the parasites soon enough you can cure all cancer. She backs up her argument with 100 case histories.

Obesity increases your probability of getting cancer. You should know about the dreaded fat virus. Adenovirus 36 may hold the secrets to those stubborn pounds that will not go away. It has long been suspected that either a virus or parasite often causes obesity. The pathogen causes people to store excess fat.

Doctors Nihil Dhurandhar and Richard Atkinson, at the University of Wisconsin Medical School, have come up with startling evidence that proves an inhuman terrorist is at work.

Two studies showed that in many cases Adenovirus 36 is the real reason you just cannot lose weight and keep it off. One study tested 154 obese volunteers and 45 lean volunteers for Adenovirus 36 antibodies. 24 of the obese volunteers tested positive. That is about 15%. None of the lean volunteers tested positive.

The second test used animals. They injected chickens and mice with the human virus and watched to see what would happen. The infected animals began to gain fat. When the test was ended the infected animals had put on two and one half times as much fat. That's a 250% increase in fat production and storage.

The list of these hidden terrorists continues to grow. It is now linked to Alzheimer's, Cardiovascular Disease, and Autism. Will the list never stop?

WHAT NOW? **Transfer Factor to the rescue.** Antibiotics and vaccines are still weapons that can be used but only if the pathogen has been identified and is not drug resistant. The problem will only be solved when the body's own defense system is strong and educated. Nothing does this better than Transfer Factor.

Chapter 5

Arm the Immune System

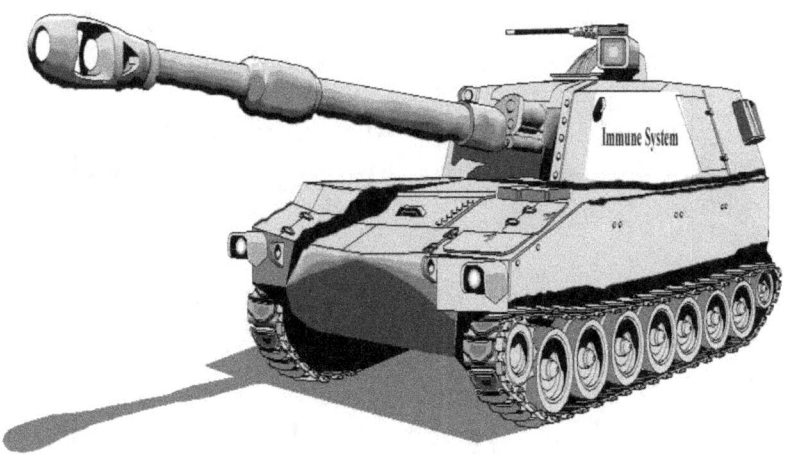

Intelligence is not enough. The world is full of brilliant, educated failures. Application and persistence will usually ultimately bring success. Intelligent, educated people, who apply themselves consistently, succeed faster and more consistently than those who do not have these gifts.

Transfer Factor educates the immune system extremely well but education is not enough. The immune system must be strong and constantly vigilant if it is to defeat the inhuman terrorists. The immune system must have sufficient troops, which we call Immune Cells (T-Cells, NK Cells, Macrophages, etc.) to carry out the instructions given directly or indirectly by the transfer factors.

Transfer Factor does strengthen the immune system better than other natural immune system boosting supplements that I have found. It is also a great team player. It makes allies of other supplements.

The following chart shows how it stands up to the competition. It also shows how well it works with its competition.

Immune Booster Comparison

15%	Noni (Morinda Citrifolia)
15%	Aloe Vera Concentrate
16%	Endocrine System Formula
21%	Phytonutrient with Garlic
23%	Bovine Colostrum
28%	Cordyceps Formula
42%	Shiitake Mushrooms
43%	Echinacea
48%	Plant Polysaccharide
49%	IP6
103%	Transfer Factor
248%	Transfer Factor & Allies

Percent rise in NK Cell activity over baseline

Noni and Aloe Vera are both known worldwide for their immune system boosting abilities. Their reputation is well deserved. A 15% increase in NK cell activity makes a big difference in the destruction of inhuman terrorists. You could get well days sooner. If a 15% increase makes a difference what would a 103% or 248% increase do?

Transfer Factor from Colostrum alone can boost NK activity by 103%. When it teams up with its best allies the increase in NK activity is 248%.

New studies done by the Russian Academy of Medical Science show that combining Transfer Factors from Colostrum and egg yolks gives an even greater boost, 287%. This blend, along with the allies, delivers a whooping 437% increase in NK cell activity. These test results were achieved after 48 hours of using the product.

When the United States launched its war against Terrorism in October of 2001, we soon discovered that there were many sympathetic, helpful allies. Some of the allies have not always, or even historically, been allies. We also discovered that not all so-called allies are consistently dependable. We were pleased to learn that some allies are always there when help is needed.

Since the extraction of Transfer Factor from Bovine Colostrum and Egg Yolks, many supplements have been tested to discover which would work best with Transfer Factor. Some supplements that did a good job of immune boosting, by themselves, did not make a big difference when added to Transfer Factor. Some made a dramatic difference.

The allies that I believe have delivered most consistently are as follows. They are listed alphabetically, not in order of importance. I do not know if anyone knows which is most important. It may vary from person to person. Here is the list: Agaricus Blazeii, Beta-Glucan from Baker's Yeast, Beta-Glucan from Oats, Cordyceps sinensis, IP-6 (Inositol hexaphosphate), Maitake Mushroom extract, Mannans (from Aloe Vera leaf), Olive Leaf Extract, Shiitake Mushroom, Soya Bean Extract, and Zinc.

Who are the Allies?

Agaricus Blazeii is a mushroom said to fight Cancer. In a study done on guinea pigs at the Medical Department of Tokyo University, the National Cancer Center Laboratory and Tokyo College of Pharmacy **Agaricus** outperformed all other mushrooms tested to fight cancer. The cure rate for the cancer tested was 99.4%.

Beta-Glucan has been studied as much as any immune booster in recent years. Harvard, Tulane, and the US Armed Forces are just a few of the institutions that have studied it. The tests always come out positive. This ally stands with us every time. The peer-reviewed studies all say it is both safe and effective in boosting the immune system.

Beta Glucan stimulates both the production and activity of macrophages. Macrophages are soldiers who roam our bodies consuming inhuman terrorists and cleaning up the trash they leave behind.

There are several sources of Beta Glucan. There is a war of words debating which is the best source. The top two contenders, Brewers Yeast and Oats, both have qualities that are unique. I think it is a good idea to have both forms of Beta Glucan as allies.

Beta Glucan is best known for: anti-oxidant properties, radiation protection, tissue repair and immune system boosting.

The people who need it most are those who: Travel on airplanes, have x-rays or mammograms, live or work near high tension power lines, work on computers, or are exposed directly or indirectly to the sun. I think that takes in most, if not all, of us.

Cordyceps is native to the highlands of China, Tibet, and Nepal, above 10,000 feet. It is growing very scarce in the wild but, fortunately, it has been successfully cultivated. It is now grown in higher elevations around the world. Cordyceps sinensis is the proper name, though in China it would more likely be called Caterpillar Mushroom, Winter Worm, or Summer Grass.

The mushroom Cordyceps became popular after a group of Chinese runners broke nine world records in a single meet in Germany. Their coaches gave the credit to "The Caterpillar Mushroom". It soon became a leading sports supplement because it helps increase energy levels, endurance, and stamina.

Cordyceps sinensis is a highly valued medicinal mushroom in both classical Chinese medicine and modern Western medicine. Medically Cordyceps is used primarily to build and support the immune system.

Here is a small list of conditions said to improve with the use of Cordyceps sinensis: arrhythmia, arterial-sclerosis, cancer, chronic fatigue, cirrhosis, coronary heart disease, flabby waist, impotence, nephritis, nephropathy, respiratory conditions, rheumatoid arthritis, and senile disorders. There are those who make anti-aging claims for this supplement. It is proven to increase life expectancy.

IP6 (Inositol Hexaphosphate) is a derivative of the B-Vitamin Inositol. In his book *IP6* Dr. Shamsuddin makes IP6 sound like a cure all. He has studies to prove his claims.

His studies show that IP6 prevents the formation of some cancers. It has demonstrated an ability to shrink pre-existing cancers. IP6 boosts the immune system dramatically. Independent studies show that it increases NK Cell activity by 49%.

Other advantages of IP6 are that it helps lower cholesterol, reduces the risk of cardiovascular disease, including heart attack and stroke. It helps prevent kidney stones and the complications of diabetes and sickle cell anemia.

Maitake - The King of Mushrooms
Over 3,000 years ago Chinese Medicine included the use of this powerful healing agent. The Japanese discovered it about the same time. It is most used for serious degenerative conditions.

The Maitake mushroom is native to northeast Japan and China. It was first used to strengthen the body and improve overall health. Current research indicates that it may be the most potent immune system stimulator of all mushrooms. The compounds contained in it also inhibit tumor growth.

This friend is reported to be a Cancer Fighter, Blood Pressure regulator, Diabetes eliminator, and Weight controller. There are those who even claim it is an effective Aids fighter. World-renowned doctors like Dr. Hiroaki Nanda and Joan Priestley, MD have done some impressive studies using Maitake Mushrooms.

Mannans from Aloe Vera has been so widely known and studied that books have been written on its qualities. I will only give a very short summary. Mannans have an anti-inflammatory action in the body. Mannans are anti-viral and tend to modulate the activity of the immune system. This food is one of the few supplements that is absorbed intact by the pinocytotic process of the digestive tract.

Olive Leaf Extract is said to slow if not stop the duplication of infectious cells. In the Bible, Ezekiel 47:12 speaks of a tree near the Dead Sea that may have been an Olive tree, "...the fruit thereof shall be for meat and the leaf thereof for medicine." Some believe the active ingredient in the Olive Leaf is Oleuropein. It is a very bitter substance that is both anti bacterial and anti viral.

Shiitake Mushroom, also known as the Black, Chinese Black, or Forest Mushroom, is popular throughout Eastern Asia. It ranks number one of all edible mushrooms in Japan.

"When in doubt try Shiitake Mushroom!" has been a part of traditional medicine in Asia for thousands of years. Studies show that this friend of the healthy body alliance is useful in the prevention of cerebral hemorrhagic strokes, lowering cholesterol levels, regulating blood pressure, has anti-tumor, anti-viral qualities, and it boosts immune system activity. Those who use it say it is both a tonic and a stimulant.

The **Shiitake** Mushroom, in Latin *Lentinula edodes*, is the lover's mushroom. It has a delicious smoky flavor and is a gentle aphrodisiac when eaten alone. It exerts a greater influence when eaten with meat. Its influence is even more greatly enhanced when it is taken with wild game.

Zinc is usually an ally but in large quantity is an enemy. Zinc is universally accepted as a protector of the Immune System. Study after study shows effectiveness at increased immunity, preventing some forms of blindness, protecting against cancer, speeding wound healing, increasing male potency and sex drive, protecting the prostate, and the treatment of acne. It is necessary for proper taste, smell and vision. It has anti-inflammatory qualities that make it a friend of arthritis sufferers.
Significant Zinc deficiency in developed countries is rare but moderate to severe deficiencies do pop up occasionally.

The Doctors' Vitamin and Mineral Encyclopedia, claims Zinc has a competitive nature and competes with Copper for absorption. If you take more than 30 mg of Zinc it is a good idea to take a Copper Supplement. Tests show that if Zinc is taken in quantities of 150 mg or more it interferes with the production of HDL, the good cholesterol. Zinc is a great immune system booster when taken in small to moderate amounts but it suppresses the immune system when taken in mega doses. Safe levels are 30-50 mg per day. Any time you take more than 30 mg of Zinc a copper supplement is recommended.

Part Two
Stories of Inhuman Terrorists Defeated or Contained

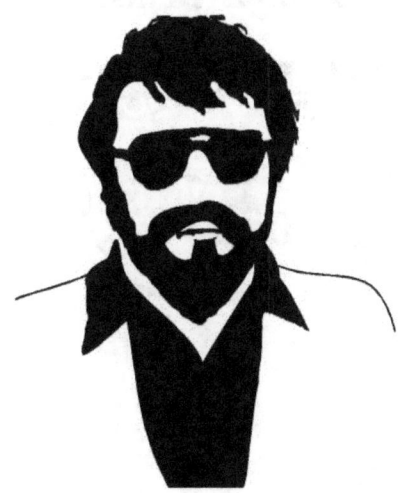

The stories used in this section are true. Most of the names have been changed to protect the privacy of those who willingly shared their experiences.

Chapter 6
Acne

Alias Zit Face

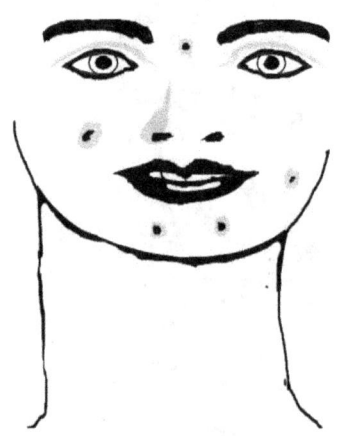

Zit Face is one of the most feared of the inhuman terrorists. It is not the most dangerous in the sense of being life threatening. It is a self-esteem destroyer. Acne usually attacks teenagers but has been known to attack humans of all ages.

Master herbalist Dr. William Horish claims, "A pimple is nothing more than a bowel movement through the skin." He notes that pimples and blackheads are one way the body eliminates toxins. These toxins often give aid and shelter to the terrorist called Acne.

One of the first steps in eliminating this vile villain is to get rid of its support structure. Once this is done, the immune system, trained and reinforced by Transfer Factor, will make short work of old Zit Face.

Step one is clean the skin with a purifying cleanser. You want one that dissolves excess oils.

Step two, clean your colon using a high quality fiber system combination and a cleansing tea. A blend of Senna Leaf, Stevia Leaf, Cinnamon Bark, Buckthorn Bark, Ginger Root, Natural Apple Flavor, Orange Peel, Green Tea, Bitter Orange, Echinacea, Roibos and Astragalus Root would be a great tea for life.

Marsha had been searching to get rid of the terrorist Acne. She felt like she had tried everything. She took antibiotics for five years but Zit Face got through her security. She said that the antibiotics helped but only removed 80% of the problem. When she stopped the drugs the problem came back.

At last she called on Transfer Factor for help. The results were pleasing. She gave this report, "After 6 weeks on Transfer Factor my acne completely cleared up."

Her dermatologist wanted information on Transfer Factor. There is a ground swell of dermatologists recommending Transfer Factor to their patients. The number grows as information spreads.

Some people get rid of Acne with colon cleansing and Transfer Factor. Others need Transfer Factor plus allies. Chickweed is often a great ally against Zit Face.

Chapter 7
Arthritis
Inflictor of Pain

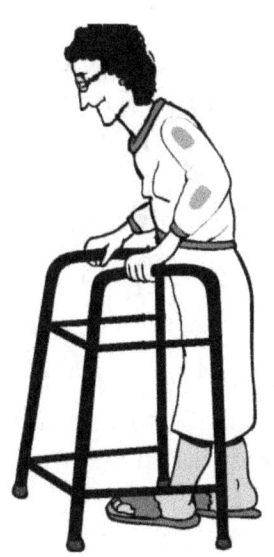

One name, many Inhuman Terrorists. The New American Medical Dictionary and Health Manual defines Arthritis simply as, "Inflammation of a joint." But it is very complex. There are many kinds of Arthritis. It comes in a host of forms. Many have been classified and others are yet to be found. Some of the more common forms are:

Acute. It is joint inflammation. It comes on fast if not suddenly. Common symptoms are heat, pain, redness, and swelling.

Allergic. Joint inflammation that follows contact with a substance to which the patient is allergic.

Degenerative. This type of Arthritis is accompanied by the loss of cartilage around the joints. Stiffness and deformity follow.

Gouty. Usually only affects one joint at a time. It is caused by an upset in uric acid balance and metabolism.

Rheumatoid. It is one of the more common chronic forms of joint inflammation. It usually affects several joints at the same time. There is usually pain and some limitation of movement. scientist do not know which inhuman terrorist causes this problem but it is generally thought to have an infectious origin.

Arthritis is generally considered an autoimmune disease. That means our bodies' police force is attacking us, thinking our body parts are inhuman terrorists.

Transfer Factor fights this condition in two ways. First, it teaches the immune system what and who the real terrorists are. Second, it teaches the body not to attack itself.

There are many allies that can aid in the battle against the monsters we call Arthritis. They play dual roles. One is to minimize the damage caused when our bodies attack themselves. The other is to speed healing and reduce symptoms. The following testimonials give only a small percentage of the herbs and formulas that are available as allies.

Three years ago, Don contracted polymyositis, a very painful form of arthritis that destroys the muscles. Exercise is usually an ally to those suffering from Arthritis. It hurts but it generally makes the condition better. Because of the nature of polymyositis exercise is usually not a viable option.

Don tells how a friend introduced him to Transfer Factor and two combination supplements originally formulated to treat fibromyalgia. There is a formula to use in the daytime and one for the evening. The daytime blend is Vitamin B6, Magnesium, Malic acid, Glucosamine, Bovine Cartilage Hydrochloride, Mucopolysaccharides and Chondroitin Sulfates, MSM, Boswellia Serrata, N-acetyl Cysteine, Bromelain, L-Cysteine, Grape extract, Devil's Claw, Alpha Lipoic acid, and Boron.

The nighttime formula is a blend of Vitamin B6, Melatonin, Pregnenolone, 5HTP, Simplicifolia, Creatine monohydrate, N-acetyl Cysteine, Pau D'arco, Valerian, Kava Kava, Grape extract, and Alpha Lipoic Acid. This formula helps a person sleep so they can heal.

Don is, and will always be, grateful to his friend because the pain went away. Don had been taking the Transfer Factor and allied combinations for just over three weeks when some amazing things happened.

The pain went away. Don felt so good he had the courage to install a satellite dish on his house. He was up and down, up and down, about ten times.

You would have thought he would have been exhausted. Staying home and watching TV, scanning the new channels would have been most people's plan. But not Don, he felt so good that he went bowling that night.

Friday morning came. He awoke ready to pay the price of the previous days activities. He moved slowly at first to avoid the pain. To his surprise there was no pain. Does he like Transfer Factor and its allies? Don says, "I love it."

It's a miracle

Cheryl was diagnosed with a very aggressive form of rheumatoid arthritis about six years ago. The terrorists that attacked her body were very aggressive. Within months of being diagnosed, her pain was almost unbearable. If she sat down on anything soft she needed help to stand. She complained, "I couldn't even walk up the stairs!" Because every stair she climbed represented pain, she could tell the exact number of stairs in her house.

When she awoke in the morning she could barely stand. She was practically immobile for 15 to 20 minutes. The pain level was intense. Life was not fun. She was motivated to find a solution. She tried everything that promised help. If it came from a doctor or multi-level marketer she was open to try it. "You name it, I tried it. Nothing worked." she reported. She had the courage to keep trying when many would have given up. At last she found out about Transfer Factor and the two allies mentioned in the previous story.

Cheryl was motivated. She would have been happy for even a night without pain so she could sleep. Just the weight of her blankets would wake her up two or three times every night. Her pain was nonstop. To say she did not sleep well was a gross understatement.

She began taking the Transfer Factor and its allies. She hoped for a miracle and expected another disappointment.

Just six days into the program she awoke and realized a pleasant surprise. "Wow, I just slept through the night with no pain! No pain! **First time in six years!**", she shouted. Whether she shouted out loud or to herself I don't know, but what matters is that most days she is pain free. The swelling has gone down. She says it is **a miracle** but the truth is that Transfer Factor and its allies are just doing their job.

Some other allies in the battle against Arthritis in all its forms are: **Essential Fatty Acids**, **Cherries** (Black Cherries are best for most forms of Arthritis. All Cherries work well for gout.), **Bee Pollen, OPC's** (Both **P**ine **B**ark and **G**rape **S**eed Extracts work well. They work synergistically together.), **Aloe Vera**, and **Noni Juice**.

A combination that keeps people flexible for life is a blend of key fatty acid esters, Glucosamine and Chondroitin.

Chapter 8
Asthma
The Strangler

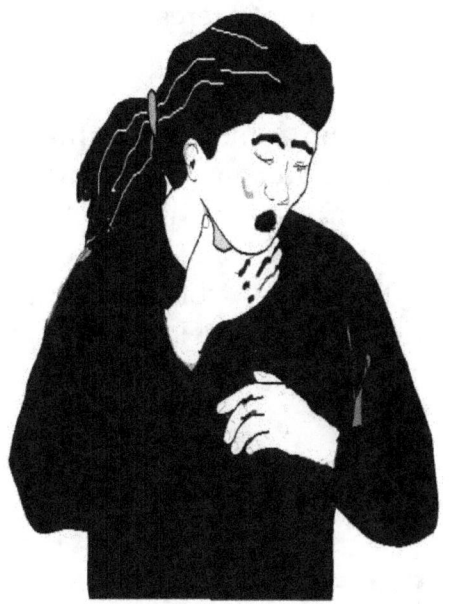

The Boston Strangler brought fear into the hearts and minds of many people especially the people of Boston. The very thought of being without air is frightening. There are people who will not cruise or ride in a boat because they fear drowning. The inhuman terrorist Asthma kills more people in the USA every year than all murders and drowning in all North America. It interferes with the lives of millions.

Those who have asthma and those who have come close to drowning understand the panic and fear associated with suffocation. When the chest is plugged up, when air will not go in or come out, when you can't breathe, you are desperate for anything that delivers relief. Nature has given us a few friends who will help. Transfer Factor is one of the best.

> **When you can't breathe, you are desperate for anything that delivers relief.**

I do not know if anyone knows the real cause of Asthma but they have some good ideas. Before I discovered Transfer Factor and its allies I frequently suffered from Asthma. Visits to the emergency room and hospital stays were a common thing for me. On one of my visits I asked why some people have Asthma and others do not. The doctor explained that there were five common forms of Asthma. One is caused by stress and a dry climate. The second is caused by stress and a damp climate. The third is caused by allergies and a dry climate. The forth is caused by allergies and a wet climate. The fifth is a combination of the other four. A new theory is that Asthma is caused by bacteria that live in the air passages and cause inflammation.

Whether the doctor was right or wrong about the causes of Asthma there is one fact we must accept. Asthma is a potentially life-threatening condition in which the victim may suffocate. Whatever the trigger is, the body attacks itself. The bronchial tubes constrict and do not allow air to go in or out. Many Asthma victims can get air in, but cannot exhale. It is very common to have a loud, wheezy noise associated with asthma.

Asthma, the Strangler, like Arthritis and MS, is a known auto-immune disorder. Transfer Factor is an immune system educator. The result is immune system modulation.

Therefore, Transfer Factor often down modulates an overactive immune system. Not everybody will get the same results. For some conditions Transfer Factor works remarkably fast. For most people, time and consistent use of the product brings the best results. The speed of transition in the following story is an exception, not a rule.

Deb had chronic Asthma. Every day of her life she had to fight for breath. Modern science and God kept her alive. She was dependent on inhalers to keep her air passages open. Three or four times a day she was forced to puff on her inhalers. She was aware of the side effects of the inhalers but they were not as bad as the side affect of not breathing.

A relative suggested she give Transfer Factor a try. He told her not to expect anything for at least 30 to 45 days. It takes time to fully educate an immune system.

To everyone's surprise Deb had marked improvement the second day on Transfer Factor. She was so improved she did not need her inhalers the whole day.

Every day for the first week Deb expected the Asthma to return. Apparently this terrorist knows when to stay away because Deb continues to breathe freely and easily. Only those who have had a challenge breathing know what a blessing it is to breathe without effort. The relative asked me to pass this message on, "Don't delay in telling those people you care for about this incredible life changing substance! Do it today!

There are a few other allies that often help Transfer Factor defeat Asthma. They include Bee Pollen, Lobelia, Noni Juice, and **Pine B**ark and **Grape Seed** Extracts

Chapter 9
Autism
It Silences Its Victims

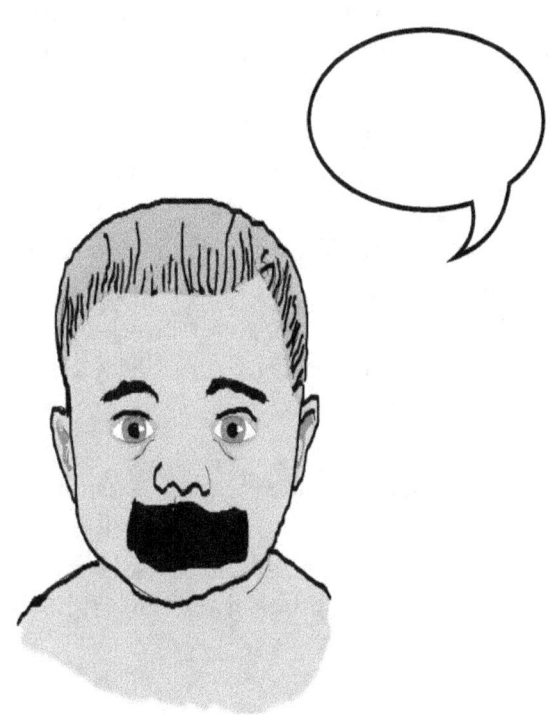

Infantile Autism, sometimes called Kanner's syndrome, is one of the vilest of terrorists because it attacks babies. It usually shows up while the baby is less than a year old. It never shows up after a child is 30 months old. We do not know all the forms this terrorist takes to enter and attack babies but there are some strong indications. The terrorist known as Rubella is most frequently suspected. It is believed that the virus gets to the child either because its mother got Rubella while she was pregnant with this child or the child was given a measles, mumps, and rubella vaccination.

This villain is between two and four times as likely to attack a boy rather than a girl. It is characterized by extreme aloneness or apparent lack of attachment, insistence on sameness, insomnia, repetitive limb movements, and strong attachment to familiar objects. Often there is difficulty with speech. If they speak at all they usually use the word "you" in place of "I" and "me". These children have uneven intellectual development in most cases. One parent told me, "My boy is smart, he is just locked in a cage."

Allies like Bee Pollen and quality multi-vitamin/minerals have long been known to aid victims of autism. But they have only made a little difference. Seldom have they brought about a dramatic change.

Transfer Factor makes a difference. Recently, a group of researchers performed a closely scrutinized study of the affect of Transfer Factor on Autism. Could Transfer Factor really bring the usually sluggish immune systems of Autism victims to life? Could their systems be educated? Would it make a difference in their mental function?

The test delivered great results. As expected, the immune system began to function better. Here are the results. I suspect they were unexpected. Out of 22 autistic patients 21 improved. Ten, almost half, achieved adequate mental and emotional improvement to enrol in mainstream schools. This was an almost unbelievable achievement.

Dr. Dave was concerned about the low immune systems of 4 or 5 victims of Autism. They seemed to get every bug that came along. He decided to test the effect of Transfer Factor. He got more than expected.

As he anticipated, the immune function improved in every case. What surprised him were the results that he did not expect. In his own words,
"...interestingly, all have shown improved communication skills, better interactive skills, and less self-stimulatory behaviour." Needless to say, all of the parents are absolutely delighted. The only ones complaining are the inhuman terrorists.

Mack's 4-year-old son suffers from Autism. Mack and his wife believe in vitamins and supplements and have always given their child everything they thought he needed. Their son, like many others, also had mercury poisoning.

The boy was receiving both mercury toxicity and behavioural therapy. The results were limited till Mack and his wife learned about Transfer Factor and began feeding it to their child. They thought they noticed marked improvement. It was confirmed when they held a birthday party for their son. Several parents commented on how amazed they were with the boy's improvement.

Speaking of his son with Autism, Mack said that his son had gone from being the most often sick person in the family to the least often sick.

Mack and his whole family now take Transfer Factor. Mack was so impressed with the results his family had that he chose to sell Transfer Factor.

In Hawaii, an eleven year old boy, for the first time, was able to tell his parents about a problem on the school bus after eating Transfer Factor for just a few months. When the parents added a targeted Transfer Factor the skills trainer noticed a positive difference the first day. The boy is now 12 and mainstreaming three of his classes. They are easy classes.

Chapter 10
Bronchitis
The Gunk Men

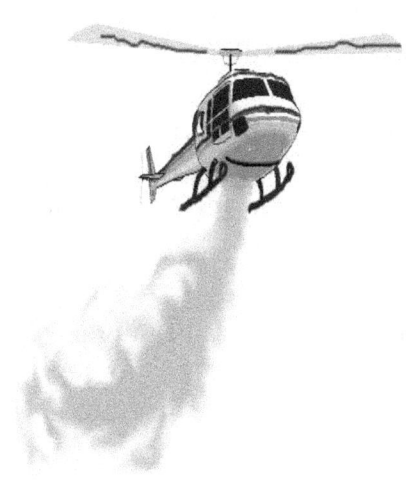

The terrorists collectively known as The Gunk Men cause a condition known as Bronchitis. Bronchitis is nothing more or less than inflammation of the bronchial tubes. It can be caused by asthma, bacteria, viruses, mold or air pollution. Its symptoms are much the same as Asthma. In fact, Asthma and Bronchitis often work together to make your life miserable. One tends to cause the other.

Bronchitis often starts out as a cold or flu. It sets up a condition that makes you more vulnerable to Pneumonia.

Bronchitis is usually accompanied with thick mucus that can block airways. These terrorists fill your Bronchi with gunk, which you must cough up. You are faced with the painful decision whether to swallow it or spit it out.

Damage to the lungs and voice are common with chronic Bronchitis because of the pressure applied both to the lungs and vocal cords with persistent coughing which goes on for years.

A Bronchitis cough is often very loud. It can be embarrassing at church, movies, plays, or any occasion where one is expected to be quiet.

Unlike Asthma, Bronchitis is not generally considered an autoimmune condition. The theory is, "Get rid of the inhuman terrorist that causes Bronchitis and the Bronchitis goes away. If I were fighting Bronchitis I would take Transfer Factor plus allies. (Agaricus Blazeii, Beta-Glucan from Baker's Yeast, Beta-Glucan from Oats, Cordyceps sinensis, IP-6 (Inositol hexaphosphate), Maitake Mushroom extract, Mannans (from Aloe Vera leaf), Olive Leaf Extract, Shiitake Mushroom, Soya Bean Extract, and Zinc.)

The mucous associated with Bronchitis can be reduced by taking digestive enzymes and friendly bacteria. The blend of enzymes I would use is a combination of Amylase, Invertase, Glucoamylase, Proteases, Cellulase, Peptidase FP, alpha-Galactosidase, and Lipase. I would also take the following friendly bacteria: Lactobacillus acidophilus, Lactobacillus casei, Bifidobacterium bifidum, Bifidobacterium longum, Lactobacillus plantarum, and Lactobacillus reuteri.

This blend of digestive enzymes and probiotics (friendly bacteria) has the side affects of improving digestion and absorption. It also protects the body against certain inhuman terrorists that live in the digestive tract.

Noni has a good reputation as an ally against Bronchitis.

A blend of the following herbs helps clear breathing passages and delivers symptomatic relief while you wait for Transfer Factor plus its allies to eliminate the Bronchitis. The herbal blend is Boneset, Fennel, Horseradish, Mullein, and Horehound.

Nadine suffered from chronic bronchitis for fifteen years before she discovered Transfer Factor. She had an embarrassing cough that was always there. At night her own coughing would often awaken her.

The lack of sleep caused by the coughing may have been responsible for her constant fatigue and frequent migraine headaches. Her regular sinus infections and allergies did not make things any better.

Nadine was developing joint pain and a sense of overall weakening when, at last, she discovered Transfer Factor.

I learned about Nadine's plight after she had been taking Transfer Factor for eight months. Did it make a difference? Nadine says, "I am a new person. I feel like Transfer Factor saved my life." The bulk of her health problems are a thing of the past.

Chapter 11

Cancer
This Terrorist is a Real Crab

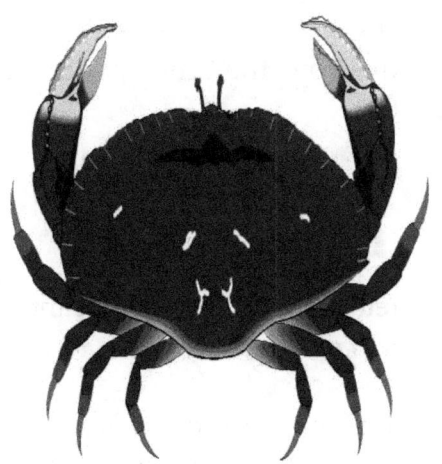

Cancer is one name given to a large group of deadly inhuman terrorists. The many types of Cancer, for the most part, operate the same way. Step by step they take over and destroy the body. Untreated it is usually fatal.

The six insidious steps of Cancer terrorists are:

> **First,** invade the cell and destroy normal controls. On a cellular level, this is the equivalent of infiltrating an organization and getting a key leader hooked on both heroin and crack cocaine.

> **Second,** stimulate unregulated cell growth.

> **Third,** destroy the ability of the cells to differentiate.

> **Fourth,** empower cancer cells to invade local tissues.

> **Fifth,** metastasize or spread cancer to other organs or parts of the body.

> **Sixth,** after months or years of terrorizing and torturing its victim this heartless inhuman terrorist kills its host.

In the 1960's one in every five people got cancer. 1 in 8 died of cancer. Today more than 1 in 3 will have cancer in their lifetime. Clearly, this villain has been very successful and is getting more aggressive. Conventional medicine has been unsuccessful in slowing the spread of this killer. If cancer continues to spread at its current rate, everyone will have cancer in his or her lifetime. That is 100% of the population. Can this terrorist be stopped? I believe it can if we stop putting cancer-feeding substances in and on our bodies. Educating our immune systems with Transfer Factor is a must.

Because this terrorist is so successful I would always use Transfer Factor plus its standard allies to defeat this villain. A recent closely controlled study by the Russian Academy of Medical Science shows why. The study compared the effectiveness of the chemotherapy drug Interleuken-2 with the NK Cells of a person taking Transfer Factor plus its allies in killing Cancer cells. The drug killed 88% of the Cancer cells. Transfer Factor and allies empowered NK Cells to kill 97%. The Transfer Factor and allies had no negative side affects, which cannot be said of the Doctors big gun, Interleuken-2. Remember, this study was a test tube study. In the human body there are many variables.

In addition to the usual allies, I would call in some Cancer specialists. A powerful antioxidant is a must. I would likely use a blend of **Pine Bark** and **Grape Seed** extract or Grape Seed combination that contains Trans-Resveratrol. These extracts contain Proanthocyanidins (OPCs), which are thought to prevent oxidative damage to cellular membranes.

Because of the drugs used and chemical changes that occur when someone gets Cancer, two problems often show up. The first terror conspirator is the death of friendly necessary bacteria. The second conspirator is insufficient digestive enzymes. Digestive Enzymes, Probiotics (friendly bacteria) are a good idea. They make it possible for you to get the most out of both food and supplements.

It is important to take a Multivitamin/Mineral supplement that is both bio-active (will work in the body) and bio-available (is easily absorbed in the right parts of the body). Many Multivitamin/Mineral supplements on the market are neither bio-active nor bio-available. The little extra money you pay for quality is money well spent.

Essiac Tea has turned the tide in many battles against cancer. This blend of Turkey Rhubarb Root, Sheep Sorrel, and Burdock Root came to us out of Canada courtesy of Rene M. Caisse who learned its secrets from an Indian medicine man. Cassie's Tea is often a lifesaver.

If you have been singled out by cancer, your physical condition could discourage the attack. The stronger your body, the less likely you are to be a victim. If you are attacked, a strong body could make the difference between life and death.

I would use Bee Pollen both as a preventative and as a warrior. Pollen is rich in enzymes and phytonutrients that could make a difference.

A Death Defying Study

Dr. Darryl See, M.D. conducted a study on twenty terminal cancer patients. Twelve were men and eight were women.

All of the patients had advanced cancer and were only expected to live 3.7 months. The Oncologist had given up hope. These people were tactfully told to go home and die. Stop spending money on treatments that will not make a difference. The average age of this group was just under 50. They had a lot of life yet to live.

> **Twenty sentenced to death by evil cancer terrorists.**

Each patient in the study agreed to take 9 capsules a day of Transfer Factor plus a group of allies: Beta-Glucan, Cordyceps, IP6, Maitake Mushroom, Mannans, Shiitake Mushroom, Thymus Complex, and Zinc. In addition, they called in the help of Digestive Enzymes, Probiotics, (friendly bacteria) Multivitamin/Mineral supplements, and proven antioxidants in standard quantities.

Eight months later, (four months after they were all expected to die,) 16 of the patients were alive. Transfer Factor plus its allies cannot save everyone, but 4 out of 5 is not a bad record. Of those who survived, some were in remission, some were improving, and the worst were stabilized.

Like most advanced cancer patients the immune system was suppressed. The baseline for natural killer cell function was only 6.4. Four weeks into the program the count was up to 25.7. Six months later it was 27.6. A 400% increase in NK Cell function is significant.

> **Four months after they were all expected to die, 16 of the patients were alive. Transfer Factor does not save everyone, but 4 out of 5 is not bad .**

It is wonderful to beat Cancer just when Cancer thinks it is about to kill another victim. It is better to beat this terrorist before it does major damage. Best is to never let Cancer in. Keep Cancer out by eating a variety of fresh fruits and vegetables. You want more vegetables than fruit. Raw is better than cooked unless you have a weak digestive system. Avoid any meat that is high in nitrates. Do not use personal care products that contain harmful chemicals like Propylene Glycol and Sodium Lauryl Sulfate. Get plenty of exercise, satisfying work, play, fun, water, and sleep. And take Transfer Factor and other supplements to keep the immune system at its peak.

Here are a few personal Cancer victories. Carl was 37 years old when he was diagnosed with papillary thyroid cancer. Carl did not want to believe he was a cancer victim. He wanted a second opinion. He gave his test results to new doctors. Both pathologists came back with the same verdict. Carl had cancer.

Carl was already on a nutritional program that was better than most people's. He added Transfer Factor plus allies to his daily regimen. He took the supplements consistently.

The doctors were concerned that the cancer might spread and asked for an early operation date. Just two weeks after Carl added Transfer Factor plus allies to his daily program the doctors removed his thyroid.

The doctors were stunned when they discovered the thyroid they had just removed was cancer free. Carl takes great pleasure showing people the lab results before the surgery that said he had cancer and the lab results after the surgery that said he did not have cancer.

Lung Cancer Was Just the Start
Dana believes Transfer Factor plus allies saved her life. Near the end of 1998 her life was shattered with the diagnoses of lung cancer. The doctors believed only an aggressive attack could destroy this vile terrorist. They came up with a plan. First they would simultaneously attack the Cancer with radiation and chemotherapy. Then, with a surgical strike, they would remove the tumor and the upper third of the right lung.

The attack went as planned. The expected collateral damage happened. Vomiting, severe weight loss, and hair loss accompanied the nausea and overall weakness. The bombardment lasted 90 days. Then came the surgery. The tumor and part of the lung were extracted.

Cancer is a deceptive terrorist and things are not always what they seem. The doctors thought they had won the war. They thought all the cancer had been removed. The doctors know this villain so they blasted Dana with chemotherapy for an additional 12 weeks. They considered this action a "safety measure."

The "safety measure" caused major damage. Dana became so weak that all she could do was eat and sleep. She did very little eating. All her hair fell out. Her fingernails and teeth became brittle. Nail by nail and tooth by tooth she began to lose them. Her weight dropped to 88 pounds.

Dana hoped that, as the chemo slowly cleared out of her system, she would get well. She hoped she could just make it till fall. In August, cancer made its counter attack. The lump under Dana's arm was malignant lymphatic cancer. It was everywhere. It was final stage cancer. The doctors conceded defeat. They gave up treatment.

Dana was told she had four to six months to live at best. They encouraged her do anything she really wanted to do but she was to do it fast. It was their belief she had 45 to 60 days before she became too sick or too weak to do anything. The doctors told her that she had no hope. No one in her condition with her cancer had ever lived.

Dana gave up. She mentally accepted, as fact, that she was about to die. She broke the sad news to her children. She took an aloha trip to Hawaii with all her children.

Everyone had given up. Everyone but Dana's son that is. Her son begged and pleaded for her to try Transfer Factor plus its standard allies. She took it only to make her son happy. She was convinced it was a waste of time and money.

Transfer Factor leads a new attack. This time it is not with the big guns of modern medicine. It is with an educated and empowered immune system. 30 days pass and Dana feels stronger. She is still convinced she is going to die but she persists in taking the supplements. Her appetite returns and she begins to gain weight.

Doomsday comes and passes. Seven months after starting Transfer Factor plus its allies, about the time the doctors told her she would surely be dead, they tell her a different story. The story is, "You are a living miracle. You have no signs of cancer." Dana now has hope for tomorrow.

Death Is In the Blood, Leukemia

Ian was only two years old when he was diagnosed with Acute Lymphoblastic Leukemia, a deadly cancer of the blood. Doctors came to his aid with chemotherapy. The cancer appeared to be in remission. The vile villain cancer will often appear to be defeated when in reality it has only withdrawn and regrouped. After several years the Leukemia returned with a vengeance.

The doctors responded with a bone marrow transplant. Again cancer retreated only to return. The cycle repeated itself and then the terrorist returned in a new form, Acute Myeloblastic Leukemia. This form of cancer is hard to treat and usually wins.

The doctors initiated a very toxic course of chemotherapy. Ian's immune system began to fail. He became susceptible to infectious complications. Then the doctors brought in Transfer Factor. After two months they brought in Transfer Factor's common allies and the tide began to turn.

Ian had little trouble tolerating his therapy. With the help of the doctors, Transfer Factor plus its allies, and, as the doctors said, "Higher Authority", Ian, at age 11, soundly defeated Leukemia. The last time Ian felt he should see the doctor was in November of 1999. He was thriving and healthy. His life is now as it should be.

Prostate Cancer, the Inevitable.

Health practitioners tell men that if they live long enough they will get Prostate Cancer. I disagree with that statement. Even though it is generally true, it does not have to happen. To beat this culprit you need plenty of Vitamin D in addition to the other anti-cancer allies. The best source of Vitamin D is sunshine.

John had a PSA test of 14 and was diagnosed with moderately aggressive prostate cancer. John chose not to use conventional treatment. He elected nutrition and Transfer Factor plus its allies.

After two years of Transfer Factor plus its allies the doctor was surprised when the PSA test came back at 0.1. The astounded physician could only say, "I don't know what you are doing, but keep it up." Three years later the PSA test was less than 0.1.

John is thankful for Transfer Factor plus its allies. He is also thankful he elected not to have surgery.

I could go on for pages with Transfer Factor testimonials. We could discuss breast cancer, cervical cancer, or melanoma. I wish I could say Transfer Factor Plus its allies always cures Cancer. I cannot! In fact, it is the body's own immune system, with the help of God, that cures any condition. Transfer Factor and all its many allies only give the body the knowledge and tools to fight the battle. Winning the battle is up to the individual and God.

Chapter 12
Cold Sores

No Kisses Please!

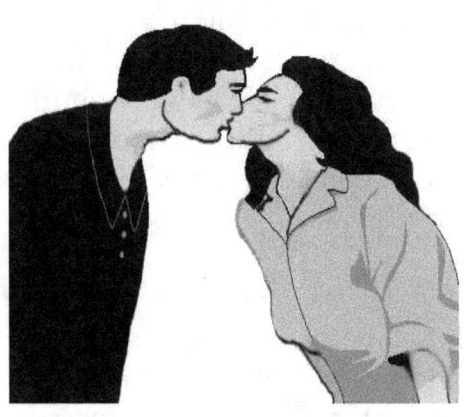

The terrorist that causes Cold Sores or Fever Blisters is Herpes Simplex 1. He is a master of disguise. The Merck manual says it is incurable. This inhuman terrorist usually launches its first attack on babies or small children. It is contagious and is spread by direct contact.

Most common treatments make the condition worse. Most authorities believe alcohol, ether, and chloroform, cause mutant and more resistant strains. The more strains of the virus you have the more breakouts you experience. Corticosteroids can spread this monster. Instead of one blister, you can have two.

This inhuman terrorist is always looking for an excuse to attack. The least little thing can bring on an outbreak. The most common causes are: a bump or scrape on the lip, dental treatment, food allergies, onset of menstruation anxiety, sunburn, or any disease or condition that produces a fever. Supplements that cause an increased metabolic rate can cause an outbreak.

Even Transfer Factor, with all its wisdom and cunning, has been unsuccessful in totally eliminating Herpes Simplex 1. Transfer Factor has been successful at making it run for cover. Most people who take Transfer Factor on a regular basis have fewer outbreaks. In one study of 22 patients, symptom-free time increased from just under 50 days to 140 days. That is a big improvement.

There is some evidence that topical application of Transfer Factor will dramatically shorten out break time. Patricia tells an interesting story. Patricia has had Cold Sores as long as she can remember. She talks about her last two Cold Sores.

Patricia explains that her friend gave her Transfer Factor. He told her that others had good results applying Transfer Factor directly on the Cold Sore. Patricia had her doubts, but she was willing to try anything that would get rid of her painful fever blisters.

She opened a capsule and dabbed some of the powder on the sore. It didn't stick very well so she did it again. It still did not stick to her satisfaction so she did it a third time and went to bed.

The next morning she was impressed to say the least. From past experience she knew this sore was just starting to grow. She expected it to grow during the night, but to her amazement it was smaller. It was beginning to heal. It made her a believer.

Unfortunately, another sore broke out about six weeks later. This time there was no delay. Patricia immediately applied the Transfer Factor. The very next morning the cold sore was in an itching healing mode. Two sores, two successes that is a good track record.

Transfer Factor can be made into a paste by adding just a few drops of water to the contents of one capsule. It is important not to smear the sore. Just dab the Transfer Factor paste directly on the cold sore. I would use a cotton swab, then discard it to avoid spreading the Herpes Virus.

If I were fighting this terrorist I would use Transfer Factor plus its allies. The addition of Olive Leaf to the list of allies will make it more powerful.

The amino acid L-Lysine and the herbs European Elderberry and Propolis will come to your aid against this villain. When taken internally, they may decrease the frequency of attacks. Chaparral may also be helpful.

Chapter 13
Diabetes
The Twin Villains

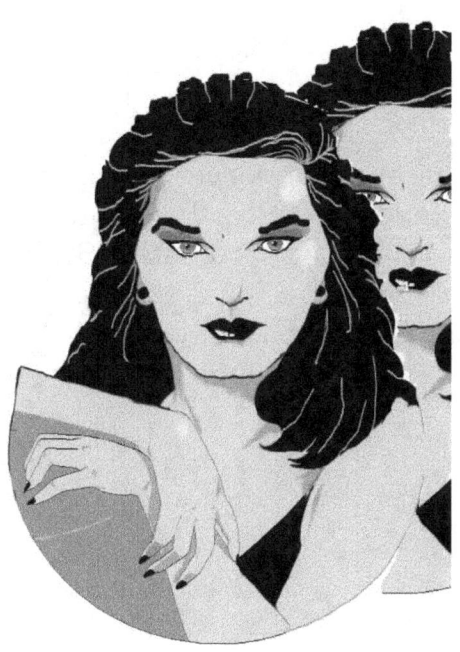

There are several terrorists who go under the name of diabetes. The two who account for 95% of all assaults are most commonly referred to as Diabetes Type 1 and Diabetes Type 2. These two villains look alike but they are each a little different. Because of advancements in medicine, diabetes is rarely directly responsible for any deaths. It is the complications of diabetes that maim and kill.

Diabetes Type 1 was once thought to be caused by heredity (a genetic flaw), or diet (too many sugars and other harmful substances). While this may still be true, modern researchers are looking to pathogens (inhuman terrorists). Some scientists suspect a bacteria or virus. Others believe the cause is a parasite. In some of my earlier Naturopathic courses the instructors taught it might be caused by a parasite.

Whatever the cause of Diabetes Type 1, the pancreas does not produce enough insulin. It usually attacks its victim before age 30. The majority of people with this condition must take insulin. Injections and insulin pumps seem to currently be the preferred delivery systems.

> ## Too little insulin is produced!

Diabetes Type 2 has most of the same symptoms and side effects as Diabetes Type 1, but the nature of the condition is very different. Victims of Diabetes Type 2 may produce plenty of insulin but the insulin receptors do not work properly. The body needs an excess of insulin in order to get enough usable insulin. It usually attacks its victims after age 30. The older a person is, the greater the chance of developing Diabetes Type 2.

The cause was once thought to be entirely diet or heredity. Today, we know that diet does play a role. Insufficient exercise plays a role. Insufficient Chromium, Vanadium, Indium, Potassium and other minerals can cause Diabetes Type 2 to attack. New evidence now points to inhuman terrorists. Is it possible that educating the immune system could eliminate the dreaded condition, known as Diabetes? Sounds like a job for targeted Transfer Factor.

We now have the means of extracting Transfer

Factors that are targeted against the terrorists that cause Diabetes. To be assured of improvement a special team of glucose allies needs to be assembled.

The strike team should include Chromium, Vanadium, Pterocarpus Marsupium, Fenugreek, Momordica Charantia, Gynema Sylvestre, Korean Ginseng, and Alpha Lipoic Acid.

Bee Pollen is a stand-alone ally. It helps prevent the complications of Diabetes.

Because of the damage done by the twin villains Diabetes Type 1 and Diabetes Type 2, Transfer Factor does not always totally eliminate these terrorists but it consistently improves the condition. Diabetes Type 2 is frequently eliminated.

Mae lives with her son and daughter-in-law. She is in her eighties and a long-time insulin user. She was taking 70 units of insulin daily when her children introduced her to the Glucose Coaching team of targeted Transfer Factors and the glucose allies. Over a six-month period of taking the Glucose TF combination, she was able to eliminate her insulin. Today, Mae's blood sugar is normal. She appears to be   completely   free   of   Diabetes.

Clark was only 11 when he was assaulted by Diabetes. As expected at this age it was Type 1. Clark was not the passive kind of person who just stood by and complained about his problem. He always strived to make life better. He was willing to try new methods of defeating the criminal that had attacked him. He joined and became president of his local chapter of Juvenile Diabetes Foundation.

He was never one to endorse anything. To get his endorsement, a product had to be very good. In 1992 he tried an insulin pump. He did endorse the insulin pump. He chose to because it changed his life and he knew it would help thousands if they used it. His name and picture have appeared nationally.

Diabetes had been working on his kidneys from the beginning but in his mid-thirties it became a problem. By the time he was 49 his kidneys were not filtering well at all. His BUN (blood urea nitrogen) tests were high. They were double normal levels. It was at this point he discovered Transfer Factor.

For 14 years the BUN readings had been high. Clark was not looking forward to his next test even though he had been using Transfer Factor. After the test the doctor called him in for a counsel. He feared the worst.

He was seated in the doctor's office, expecting tidings of doom. The doctor gave him the news, "After 14 years your kidneys are working and working well. Your BUN test is near normal." The only significant change Clark had made was adding Transfer Factor to his diet.

It was time for Clark to make another endorsement. He now endorses Transfer Factor. It changed his life.

Another victim Diabetes Type 2

Wilson was not feeling well at the first of the year. His vision would sometimes blur. He had leg cramps and a never-ending thirst. Nothing seemed to taste as sweet as it did in the past. To top it off he had psoriasis. He did not want to see the doctor but his wife insisted. She was having trouble dealing with his mood swings. Wilson consented to a physical check up.

He was shocked to discover he had Diabetes Type 2. His blood sugar count was 450. That is high. Normal blood sugar levels should be between 70 and 200. He began a program of oral medication and consistent monitoring.

After several weeks of treatment and visits to the doctor it was clear the doctor was not happy with the results. Sugar levels remained high. The medications Wilson was taking were not working as expected.

Wilson learned about Transfer Factor and began taking it. Three days passed and his blood sugar began to drop. The change was so dramatic and so sudden even the doctor was astounded. Three months after starting Transfer Factor Wilson's blood sugar was down to 110.

Wilson's Diabetes was under control but his Diabetes related psoriasis was still a problem. The flakes that fell from his head were a constant embarrassment. His skin itched most of the time. Sometimes the itch was unbearable and he would scratch till he bled. Wilson discovered Transfer Factor working with an ally named Colloidal Silver in a topical spray. The spray contained Transfer Factor and a high quality Colloidal Silver. There are many qualities of Colloidal Silver. They do not all work. The combination Wilson found was a good one.

The decision to try this combination was an easy one. Every night Wilson sprayed his head. The itching stopped almost immediately. Day by day the psoriasis began its retreat. The last time I had contact with Wilson or his wife there was still some sign of psoriasis but it was mostly gone.

Chapter 14
Fibromyalgia
Master of Concealment

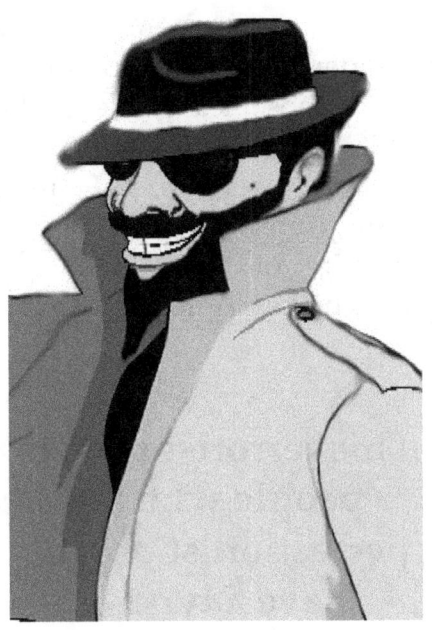

Fibromyalgia is a terrorist who has mastered concealment. The patient feels the achy pain, tenderness, and stiffness of the muscles but the doctor can't find an explanation. Fibromyalgia is a group of rheumatic disorders that are hard to define. The Merck Manual refers to them as nonarticular (unclear). The terrorist goes after women most of the time. It seems to get worse when the victim is under stress or when the baffled doctor says, "It's all in your head."

This terrorist is very real and the pain he inflicts will often disable his victim. It is like an arthritis of the muscles. It prefers to prey on people who harbor anger or are under severe physical or mental stress. It either attacks those least able to handle more problems or it makes them susceptible to more problems. Dr. Rob Robertson, M.D. reports, "There have been many published reports of low Natural Killer cell activity or function in persons with Fibromyalgia." This prompted him to do a study.

> **This terrorist prefers people who are perfectionist or who have a type A personality.**

Dr. Robertson's study involved nine people with an average NK Assay Baseline of 10. The lowest was 6 and the highest was 13. Twenty is the threshold at which people become more susceptible to acute or chronic illness. Each participant was given one capsule of Transfer Factor plus its allies twice daily for 10 days. The dosage was doubled for another 10 days. The NK cell activity was assayed again after 20 days of using the products. The new average was 26.9. The new low was 19.5 and the new high was 35.5. This change represents a 248% improvement.

For years the villain Fibromyalgia has had free reign. Even diagnosing it has been a problem. Things have changed with the discovery of Transfer Factor and some of its allies. If I were battling this terrorist I would, along with Transfer Factor, take this formula: Vitamin B6, Magnesium, Malic acid, Glucosamine, Bovine Cartilage Hydrochloride, Mucopolysaccharides and Chondroitin Sulfates, MSM, Boswellia Serrata, N-acetyl Cysteine, Bromelain, L-Cysteine, Grape extract, Devil's Claw, Alpha Lipoic acid, and Boron in the daytime. At night I would take a blend of Vitamin B6, Melatonin, Pregnenolone, 5HTP, Simplicifolia, Creatine monohydrate, N-acetyl Cysteine, Pau D'arco, Valerian, Kava Kava, Grape extract, and Alpha Lipoic Acid. The advantage of the nighttime formula is better sleep. Most of the body's repairs happen when we are sleeping.

Maria was 52 years old before her doctor suggested that she take Transfer Factor and its fibromyalgia fighting allies. Her bone and muscle pain seldom stopped. She tried doctor after doctor seeking relief. She was constantly on pain medication. Because fibromyalgia is so good at concealing its identity she had received multiple false diagnoses.

In mid 1999 she found a doctor who made a correct diagnosis. Sadly, a correct diagnosis does not mean a correct treatment. She switched doctors again. This time her doctor was holistically inclined.

The doctor started her on Transfer Factor and its morning and evening allies. He also gave her Essential Fatty Acids. She started the program in July and in August she was greatly improved. After six months she is close to being pain free. On occasion she will take an Advil or an aspirin.

Maria's life has changed. She can now hug those who are dear to her without fear of pain. She smiles more and frowns less. It is amazing the difference being pain free makes. That and a good night's sleep has made Maria a new woman.

Beverly told me her story after she had been using Transfer Factor and its Fibromyalgia fighting allies for about nine months. She told a tale of pain and suffering that had lasted over twenty years.

Beverly was strong and had learned to cope with the condition until about two years before she discovered Transfer Factor and its friends. She tried many treatments and supplements but nothing seemed to help. She began a downward spiral that seemed to have no end. Day after day she endured chronic pain and fatigue. Night after night the pain kept her awake. Depression set in. Beverly was ready to break when she discovered Transfer Factor and its Fibromyalgia/Arthritis fighting friends.

She was sleeping through the night in just two weeks. After two months on the product she described herself this way, "I felt like I had just walked out of a tunnel into the light of day." Three months on the supplements and she describes herself as 95% symptom free.

Beverly cares about people. She has shared her experience with many people. Most have had the same or similar experience of great improvement. I think she enjoys telling people about Transfer Factor almost as much as she enjoyed getting well.

Chapter 15
Hepatitis C
It hides in the Blood.

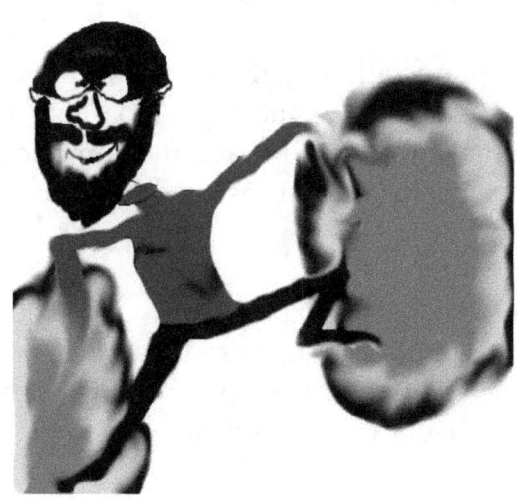

Hepatitis C is one of three common viruses we call Hepatitis. It is considered to be the most deadly form. It becomes chronic about 50% of the time. If this terrorist becomes chronic it is very hard to cure. It is often considered incurable. When this villain becomes chronic, your only real hope is an educated immune system. Transfer Factor is the only currently known method to educate it.

The onset of this villain's attack is generally milder than that of other forms of Hepatitis but the long-term damage is usually greater. About 80% of all cases of Hepatitis C come from blood transfusions. The balance usually comes from contaminated needles or sexual intercourse.

Jim is a young father with small children. He had not had success treating Hepatitis C with conventional medicine. In fact, the complications of the drugs were almost as bad as the terrorist, Hepatitis C.

He suffered digestive problems, acid reflux, and fatigue. Bowel problems were simply a way of life. He either had constipation or diarrhea. Most commonly he endured diarrhea.

Jim could see that he was losing the battle with this terrorist and was looking for a better way to fight it. He had tried several supplements but none of them had any effect. He saw an ad for a form of Transfer Factor that came with its standard allies. He thought, "I have tried everything else, why not this?"

Hepatitis C was launching a new offensive about the time Jim found Transfer Factor plus its allies and he was extremely nauseated and feeling very sick.

Transfer Factors counter offensive went slow at first. Jim said, "I just kept taking it and taking it..." Slowly he began to get better. The fatigue was the first to go. On many previous days he could not get out of bed, but after Transfer Factor, he felt like getting up. His stomach settled and he began to eat again.

Jim started cutting back on the medicine to control his bowels and acid reflux. He didn't need it any more. He began to drive and mow the lawn. Friends noticed a difference in his appearance. His liver enzymes dropped from 300 down to 194.

At this point, the war is not over but Jim is winning. He only made one mistake. When he started to feel better, he quit taking Transfer Factor. Hepatitis C came back with a furry. Jim renewed his supply and began taking the supplements again. It was not long till he was in charge again. Jim will not make the mistake of not taking Transfer Factor again. Jim took 2 capsules 3 times daily.

Chapter 16
HIV - Aids

The Defense Destroyer

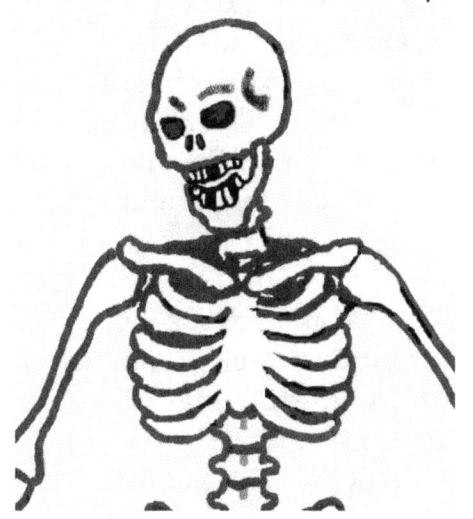

Aids is caused by a virus known as **HIV.** It spreads, primarily, through sexual contact. It can be transmitted through any body fluid. It is most prevalent among male homosexuals. Sexually active people who have frequent partners are at the greatest risk. People who require frequent blood transfusions are also high risk. Before the cause of Aids was known and because screening blood for HIV was not perfected, Aids was often spread by blood transfusion. Today this is less likely to happen.

This deadly terrorist works slow and insidiously. It eats away at the immune system day after day. People have harbored this terrorist for ten years or longer and not known it. Aids does not kill people. It is the other inhuman terrorists who take advantage of the body's compromised immune system who do the killing. Pneumonia and cancer are often the villains who take credit for the kill.

With this virus, the immune system drops and the white blood cell count drops till the body is incapable of defending itself. Modern science has been unsuccessful in stopping Aids. There have been some drugs that appear to slow it. There are also drugs that fight the opportunistic terrorists. No drug to date has been successful in curing Aids.

HIV has been so successful because of its ability to hide. It goes after the very immune system that is looking for it. If the immune system recognized this terrorist as an enemy, it could destroy it. Transfer Factor plus its allies can educate and strengthen the immune system.

Benny has Hemophilia. He has received transfusions of clotting factors since he was small. Somewhere along the line, the HIV virus smuggled itself in during a transfusion.

Benny had been on several conventional treatment regimens to stop or slow HIV. None of them appeared to work. He had side effects from most of them. His future looked dim.

He discovered Transfer Factor about the same time the doctors came up with an experimental treatment plan. He decided to do both.

Benny and those directing his quest for health suggested he take Transfer Factor plus its allies in massive quantity. He took 6 times the recommended amount of Transfer Factor and 3 times the recommended amount of the allies.

He had been on the program about 5 months when he discovered he was winning the war. He went in to see if the program was working as well as he thought it was. Everyone was surprised by the zero viral count. His CD4 count was 475 and improving. This was considered close to being a miracle. The normal CD4 count is 1000 to 1300.

Has Benny won the war? No one knows because HIV is a master of concealment. But it looks like HIV has lost. Three months after the zero viral count he repeated the test. The count was still zero. The CD4 count was up to 525.

The last report I received, the viral count was still zero and the CD4 count was normal. From rapid decline to apparently well in less than a year is truly a defeat for HIV.

Who gets the credit? The doctors may give it to the experimental treatment. The herbalists may give it to Transfer Factor plus its allies. It may have been a combination of factors. We will never know for sure but I think, along with Benny, that God and Transfer Factor plus its allies are the real heroes.

Chapter 17
Thyroid
The Regulator

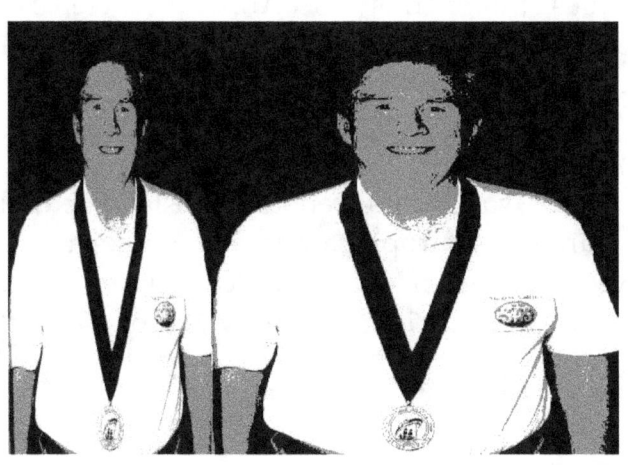

The Thyroid gland is located near what we call the Adam's Apple. It plays many roles but its major function is the control of our metabolism. When it works right we feel good and usually look good. When it overworks we lose weight, get nervous and jittery, and suffer extreme fatigue. When it under works we usually get tired and fat. Often people with under active thyroids develop goiters. These are lumps or growths. In the past they have not been associated with inhuman terrorists. Today there may be a terrorist connection.

People are taking Transfer Factor, educating their immune system and the goiters are going away. In the past I have changed the names to protect the privacy of people who willingly shared their testimonies. But in this case Annette Howell is so excited she wants everyone to hear the story in her own words.

"Hello, I am Annette Howell from Sanger, CA (near Fresno) and was introduced to Transfer Factor by Willa Duree, a Chiropractor in the Sanger area. I have been on the product a little over one month and want to say that it has helped me sooooo much.

I have had a sore throat since childhood, and now even in my 50's, I am on the verge of a sore throat every day. I have learned to control it by not stressing, etc. Since taking Transfer Factor, 3 times a day mostly, my throat does not hurt. The swelling, redness, and pockets inside the tonsil area have reduced to almost normal.

My glands on the side of the neck have always been sore to the touch, now they are not. I have had a goiter for over 20 years. Now it has almost shrunk to nothing. It was the size of a small lemon before I started Transfer Factor. Lastly, my skin (age spots) have faded away and look like freckles."

Gail had been on medication for several years to control the size of her goiter. The medication helped but failed to eliminate the problem. She could always see or feel the goiter.

Because Gail wanted to be healthy and have a strong immune system she started taking Transfer Factor. She had no hopes or expectations that it would have any affect on a goiter. The change in her goiter came as a complete surprise.

Four days after starting a Transfer Factor program Gail's life began to change. Our hero had begun an assault on the goiter. You could see that the enlargement on her neck was in retreat.

In just ten days Transfer Factor's goiter invasion appeared to be over. All signs of the goiter were gone. Gail could neither feel nor see it.

Will everyone get the same results as Gail and Annette? I can't say. It is the body's own immune system that wages and wins the fight. Transfer Factor supplies intelligence and support. It does not fight the fight.

The allies most likely to help build a strong healthy thyroid are Norwegian Kelp, Bladderwrack, and all dark leafy green vegetables. Raw vegetables are better in most cases.

Chapter 18
It Aims for the Heart but Has No Love

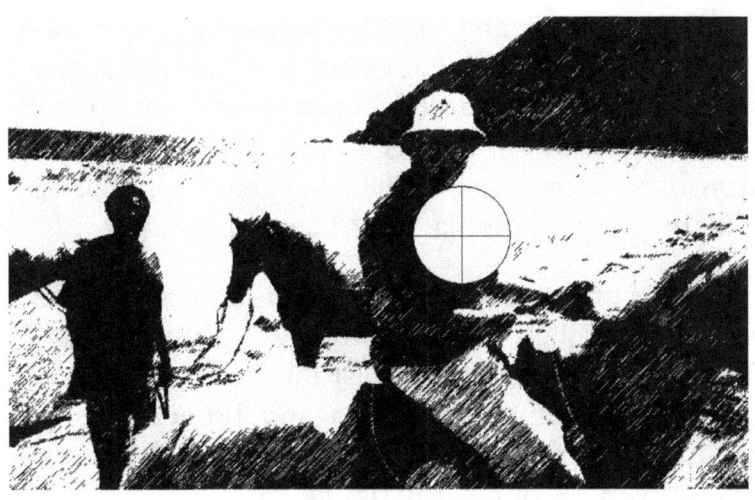

Heart disease, the villain that killed both of my parents in their forties, may be caused by a bacteria. Cardiovascular disease kills more men and women in the United States of America and Canada than any other cause. It is the leading killer in all ethnic groups. More than 960,000 Americans die of cardiovascular disease every year. Cancer is gaining on it but it is still the number one killer. Heart disease accounts for 40% of all deaths in North America.

Your doctor may tell you to eat better, lower your cholesterol level, and exercise regularly. This is still good advice. It will increase your life expectancy and quality of life but it will not ensure a life free of cardiovascular problems. Not while inhuman terrorists run free. The alleged criminal is Chlamydia pneumoniae alias C. pneumoniae.

Solid circumstantial evidence links arteriosclerosis, sometimes called atherosclerosis, to C. pneumoniae. The rap sheet of this terrorist includes community-acquired pneumonia, asthma and bronchitis. This villain is found in 52% of unhealthy aortic tissue and only in 5% of healthy tissue.

More damning evidence. When white rabbits received a couple of C. pneumoniae injections six out of nine, or two thirds of the rabbits, developed atheroscleroic looking changes in their aortas. It happened in two weeks or less.

Is C. pneumoniae an innocent bystander or a vile villain? You be the judge.

Carol lives in the mountains. It is a beautiful place to live but she suffered from a cardiovascular condition. In the fall she loved to walk into the hills and admire the beautiful view of the trees of every color. Unfortunately, she did not have the energy. Her legs were swollen. Life was not as good as it should have been

A friend suggested she take her cardio-targeted Transfer Factor with the right set of allies. In less than a week, the swelling in her legs was gone. She was walking endlessly to make up for lost time. She now is enjoying life to the fullest. She has both the time and energy to enjoy her beloved mountains and trees. She is very devoted to her children and grandchildren. She now has the time and energy to enjoy them.

The Vitamin allies I would use to improve cardiovascular conditions are: Vitamin A, Vitamin C, Vitamin E, Niacin, Vitamin B6, Folic Acid, and Vitamin B12. Herb, Mineral, and Supplement allies are: Magnesium, Zinc, Selenium, Copper, Potassium, Butchers Broom, Ginkgo Biloba, Hawthorn, Garlic, CoQ10, and Ginger Oil. Add the Essential Fatty Acids you will have a complete team.

This group of allies along with targeted Transfer Factors performs three major tasks in addition to educating and strengthening the immune system: 1. Promotes healthy blood flow to the whole body. 2. Protects and strengthens the heart and blood vessels. They guard against free radicals and other harmful elements. 3. Supports elasticity and flexibility of the blood vessels.

Chapter 19
Other Inhuman
Terrorists

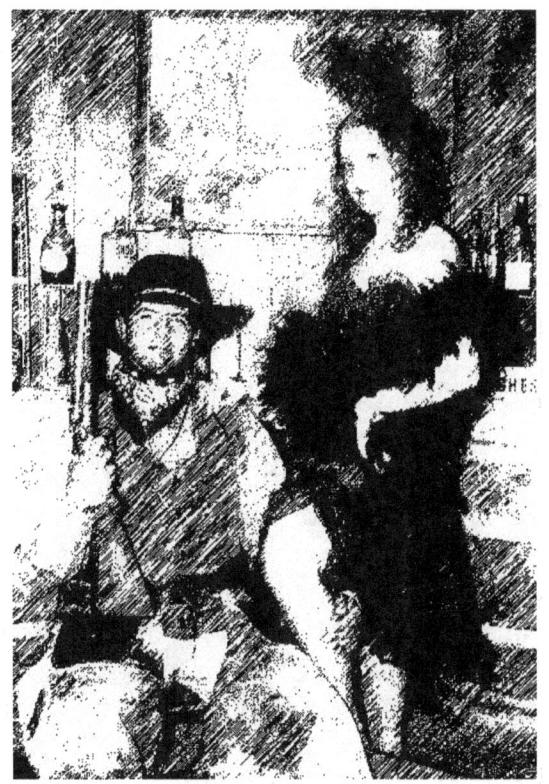

I could write chapter after chapter, condition after condition, the story would always be the same. The immune system either does not recognize the invading terrorist or it confuses a body part for a terrorist. Transfer Factor educates and supports the immune system. Transfer Factor's allies give aid and support, both to the immune system and the part or parts of the body under attack. Bodies that would have lost the fight for good health and long life win.

Here are a few more examples:

Alzheimer's and Dementia respond to memory targeted Transfer Factors and a special group of allies that frequently improve memory, emotions, and other brain functions. The allies are: Bacopa Monnieri Extract, Ginkgo Biloba Extract, Huperzia Serrata, Glycerophosphocholine, Lemon Balm Extract, N-Acety Cysteine, N-Acety Tyrosine, Soy Lecithin, and Vinpocetine.

Leilani from Oahu, Hawaii was over 90 years old when she started taking memory targeted Transfer Factor and memory boosting allies. She was suffering from short-term memory loss and Parkinson's. She took the products hoping it would help her memory. She expected no help with her shaking. Today her friends are amazed by her sharp memory but they are more impressed that she does not shake. The terrorist called Parkinson's has been defeated.

Bronchitis. Naomi had chronic bronchitis. Nothing seemed to help. After eight months of daily consumption of Transfer Factor she feels like a new person.

Ear Infections. Tommy was scheduled to have tubes put in his ears because of recurring ear infections. This terrorist had the mother taking her son to the doctor at least once a month. She discovered Transfer Factor and Tommy stopped getting ear infections. His mother said he has not been sick with anything since discovering Transfer Factor.

Flu. My daughter visited a friend in California who had the flu. The friend was the kind of person who is always willing to share. She shared the flu with my daughter. My daughter came home and shared it with me. My daughter and I were both taking Transfer Factor. We were both sick with fevers for about three days. My wife who was taking Transfer Factor plus its allies did not get sick.

The friend who gave us the inhuman terrorist had been sick a week before she infected my daughter. She was still sick a week after my daughter and I were well.

Stiff Muscles. Fran was nearing age 50. He had abused his body and it was payback time. His muscles hurt, his joints were miserable, and the pain kept him awake at night. Because he did not sleep, he was often fatigued. He had tried several supplements. Some helped more than others. None helped enough. Then he tried Transfer Factor and its Arthritis fighting allies. After four months on the program he is amazed at how good he feels.

Parkinson's Disease. Don was diagnosed with Parkinson's Disease about ten years ago. He shook, was in pain, and could not stand straight. He shook so hard that he could not write a simple letter. Life was not fun. He began taking Transfer Factor plus its standard allies. Just two months of consistent use of these inhuman terrorist eradicators and he is at least 40% better. He now works 8 hours a day. He stands straight. The pain is all but gone. The shaking is reduced and he can now write letters.

Sinus. Dale had sinus problems most of his life. By the time he reached 62, the quality of his life was dropping like a skydiver before he opens the chute. He took vitamins and other supplements but the sinus and allergy problems persisted. He started taking Transfer Factor and within hours his breathing was better. Later he added Transfer Factor plus the standard allies. Six weeks into the program and his sinus was clear. His allergies appeared to be gone.

Staph Infection. Rob had a staph infection on his arms. The Doctors had attacked it with every weapon in their arsenal but to no avail. Rob's arms would itch till he could not resist the urge to scratch. Often his arms would end up a mass of bleeding sores. In just three weeks Transfer Factor educated his immune system. The immune system eliminated the skin-harassing terrorist.

Chapter 20
Animals Are People Too

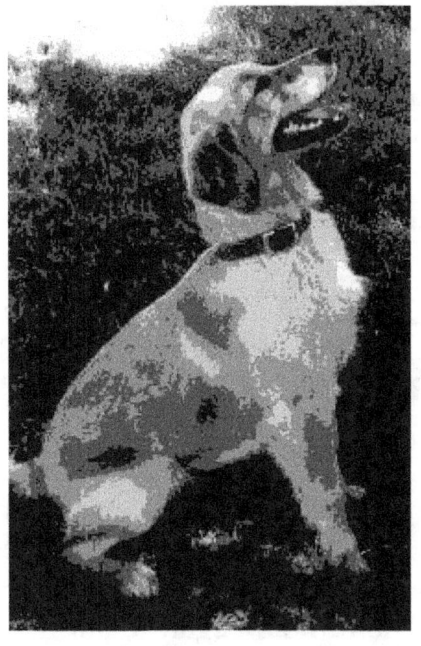

I have a daughter who is fond of telling me, "Animals are people too." She believes they have the same feelings and emotions we do even if they are not quite as smart. I cannot speak Cat or Dog so I really do not know what animals think or talk about but I do know they are often victims of inhuman terrorists.

Transfer Factor is not species specific. It works at educating the immune system of animals too.

I have included a few animal experiences suffered by some of the more common domestic animals. Here they are.

Cats

Princess had leukemia, a tumor in her mouth and a tumor on her spine. Her tail and hind legs were paralyzed. She had a poor appetite and a worse disposition.

Her veterinarian gave her 1 capsule of Transfer Factor every day. Improvement started almost immediately. Her appetite came back. She became more social. The tumors began to shrink. After five months of Transfer Factor she continues to improve. Her tail and hind legs work the way they should. Her tumors are 80% gone.

An eye-infecting terrorist attacked a Burmese cat. The Vet ran several tests but could not identify the virus villain. With salves and minor surgery the cat recovered for a few months only to have the condition return three months later.

Again the same procedure except this time a cat eye specialist was called in. This time the owner hoped for the best, only to be disappointed. Hundreds of dollars, later the terrorist returned again.

This time the owner gave the cat Transfer Factor. The cat got well on its own. It will likely stay well if the owner continues to give the cat Transfer Factor.

Tom was an 18-year-old cat with bad hips. His coat looked ragged. He was very much a couch cat. Tom was given Transfer Factor along with some cat supplements and in just three weeks he was climbing fences and acting in every way like a young cat.

Sally was a super feeble 17-year old cat. She had cloudy eyesight and serious respiratory problems. Sally was giving in to the relentless onslaught of the inhuman terrorists. Her owner had scheduled a date to have her put to sleep. As a last ditch effort, Sally's owner gave her Transfer Factor. Her eyesight improved and the respiratory problem disappeared. She is now a happy cat with expectations of a long life.

Dogs

Prince was an 8-year-old dog when investigation revealed a horrible terrorist called Cancer. A fast growing bone cancer had invaded him. The Vet told his owners that the dog had no chance of survival. He said that its bones would break just going up and down the stairs. The owners were ready to put him to sleep when a friend called and told them about Transfer Factor.

The dog had gotten so skinny it was just bones and fur. The owners gave him two capsules of Transfer Factor every day for about two months. Prince regained the weight he had lost. He began to walk and run normally. His owners thought he no longer needed the Transfer Factor so they stopped giving it to him. The cancer returned and the terrorist rejoiced. The owners recognized their folly and gave Prince Transfer Factor again. The dog now appears well in every way. We will soon have x-rays to prove the cancer is gone.

Distemper is an inhuman terrorist that is often fatal when it attacks dogs. If the dog starts having convulsions it is almost always fatal. Because Distemper is a virus that resembles HIV, dogs with this disease are often just put to sleep. Our new hero, Transfer Factor, may put an end to this practice. Read what Dr. Baruch Rosen, M.D. has to say, "As a physician of nearly thirty years, I was well aware that no antibiotic would protect against the ravages of viral disease, particularly canine distemper which shows similarities to HIV.

My seven-month-old, white haired Shepherd was adopted from a local shelter and was initially joyful and healthy. Within three weeks, he developed coarse bronchitis with heavy mucus drainage of the nose and eyes.

Our well-intentioned vet believed the problem to be kennel cough and started antibiotics. Over the next ten days Romeo failed to improve, but instead experienced seven hard and long grand mall seizures in one weekend, a partial paralysis of the hind quarters which made him fall flat when attempting to walk and a "spaced-out gaze" of non-recognition was often in his eyes.

Blood studies confirmed distemper and showed a white cell count (lymphocytes) of only 264, slightly more than ten percent of normal. Our vet, plus a second out-of-state consulting vet, an expert in distemper, were very sympathetic and advised me to prepare myself to euthanize Romeo.

The heartache was compounded when Chico, my thirteen-month-old Chihuahua, developed similar symptoms of hard coughing and heavy mucus drainage from the eyes. Reviewing his shot record, I learned he was mistakenly given only one distemper immunization, leaving him inadequately protected; and by licking Romeo's mucus and drinking from his water dish had contracted the infection.

Knowing little to nothing about canine distemper, I turned to the Internet and luckily stumbled onto Transfer Factor Plus, a preparation (Transfer Factor's standard allies) which enhances and stimulates the body's own immune system to fight against all pathogens, viral or otherwise. My thirty years in medicine told me this was the only solution. I hurriedly started Chico and Romeo on one cap daily, encased in one teaspoonful of raw hamburger.

Over the next two weeks all cough and mucus drainage ceased. Romeo's follow-up blood count had risen to a normal range at 2217 and he surprised the whole family by jumping a five-foot wall. He romps and plays all day long with Chico. He now responds normally to his name and appears to be his old joyful self again.

Having witnessed the recoveries of Chico and Romeo, and after further study, all family members are taking Transfer Factor Plus, one cap daily; our insurance policy to protect against a faltering immune system, the inevitable consequence of aging and exposure to environmental pollution and toxins. I fully intend to spread the word to all my colleagues and good friends."

Dr. Baruch Rosen, M.D.

Horse

Doctor Steven Slage, DVM tells a story about a young colt besieged with a joint infection. The inhuman terrorist had caused this poor animal to be lame for three days. One of the colt's hind legs was very enlarged at the hock (What would be considered the knee in humans.) The animal had a temperature of 104.5 degrees F. The normal temperature for a horse is 100.5 degrees F.

Doctor Slage recognized the danger this terrorist represented and recommended that the colt be hospitalized. The foal's owners were not in a position to pay for its hospitalization. The doctor then suggested penicillin injections once a day and three capsules of Transfer Factor three times a day.

48 hours later the colt was apparently well. It had a normal appetite and temperature and was no longer lame. The foal's owners confessed that they only gave the animal two penicillin shots. The colt did receive the full recommended amount of Transfer Factor. Another terrorist lost the battle.

Animal testimonies for Transfer Factor abound. As more and more pet owners and veterinarians discover that Transfer Factor is commercially available it will change the life expectancy of most pets.

Chapter 21
Autoimmune Disease
Terror of Terrorist

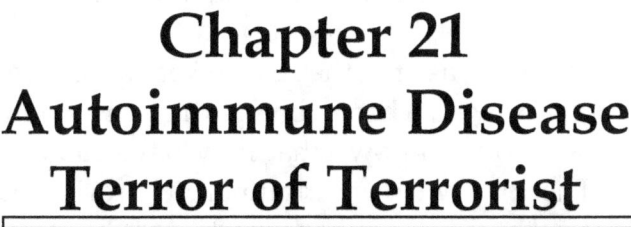

You can't see it.
Is it a Malfunction?

Autoimmune conditions may be the most feared of all conditions because, to date, modern medicine has no cures. There are treatments to mask the symptoms and make life worth living. Autoimmune conditions are conditions where the body attacks itself. No one knows for sure what causes them. They do know that if a baby is kept too clean, it is more likely to develop asthma and allergies.

Three theories as to the cause of autoimmune conditions prevail. Theory one is that it is a genetic flaw. They do not know what may have caused the flaw. Theory two is inhuman terrorist have disguised themselves as body parts and the immune system attacks the body parts thinking they are terrorists. Theory three is an immune system with nothing to attack in its formative state finds something to attack.

I do not know if any of these theories are correct or incorrect. They may all be correct or all be wrong. I do know that if the immune system were properly educated, all autoimmune diseases would cease to exist. This sounds like another job for Transfer Factor. Transfer Factor has a track record of helping the immune system discern between body parts and inhuman terrorists. I should point out that any condition branded as an autoimmune disease could be caused by an inhuman terrorist in deep cover.

Here is a list of alleged autoimmune conditions that may improve or go away with the constant intake of Transfer Factor. You will see that it is a long list.

Acute disseminated encephalomyelitis

Allergic angitis & granuloratosa (Chorg-Strauss Disease)

Anklosing spondylitis

Autoimmune Addison's disease

Autoimmune alopecia

Autoimmune chronic active hepatitis

Autoimmune hemolytic anemia

Autoimmune neutropenia

Bebcet's syndrome

Bullus pemphigoid

Dermatitis herpetiformis

Erythera nodosa

Cerebellar degneration Encephalomyelitis

Chronic bullous disease of childhood

Cicatncial pemphigoid

Classic polyarteritis nodosa

Cryopathies

Gluten-sensitive enteropathy Graft-versus-host disease

Graves' Disease

Gullain-Barre syndrome

Hashimoto's thyroiditis Hypersensitivity asolitis

Inflammatory bowel disease

Immune-mediated infertility

Insulin-dependent diabetes mellitus

Emos-Lumbert myasthenic syndrome

Isolated vasculitis of the central nervous system

Kawasaki's disease

Linear LgA disease

Multiple Sclerosis
Myasthenia gravis

Paraneoplastic pemphigus

Pemphigoid gestaionis

Pemphigus follaceus

Thyroiditis with hyperthyroidism

Type I autoimmune polyglandular syndrome

Type II autoimmune polyglandular syndrome

Primary biliary sclerosis

Psoriasis

Sclerosing cholangitis

Spidermolysis bullosa acquisita

Reactive ardrides

Rheumatoid arthritis
Sarcoidosis

Sjogren's syndrome

Stiff man syndrome

Systemic lupus erythematosus

Systemic sclerosis (scleroderma)

Taksyasa's arteritis

Temporal arteritis

Wengener's granulomatosis

As long as this list is, it is not complete. It is only a start. We may yet discover which, if any, inhuman terrorists are causing these conditions. When we do, we may find some big guns to destroy them. Till that time comes, our best allies are Transfer Factor and Bee Pollen.

Chapter 22

Attitude,
The Master
Of The Mind.

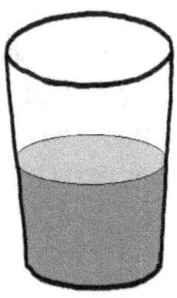

Half full or half empty?

In the beginning you were introduced to the concept of Inhuman Terrorists that invade the bodies of people, plants and animals. You learned that the body can defeat most harmful organisms or terrorists if the immune system is strong and if it recognizes the inhuman terrorist as enemies. Sometimes it needs a little help from herbs, supplements, doctors, and medication. All of these things help if the immune system is strong and educated. It is the primary job of Transfer Factor to educate. Its secondary job is to build and strengthen the immune system. As powerful as Transfer Factor is, it is useless if you do not have the right attitude.

To beat any of the most ruthless inhuman terrorist seven things are necessary. They all deal with your attitude. They are:

1. You must want to get well. It seems strange to those of us who like being well but there are those who enjoy being sick. They crave the attention and sympathy they receive when they are sick.

2. You must have hope. Holistic practitioners, herbalists, and other doctors who believe, "There are no incurable conditions, there are incurable people." are often accused of offering false hope. There is no such thing as false hope. There is either hope or no hope. The Bible tells us we should have hope. It is necessary to beat inhuman terrorists.

3. Belief is the third requirement. It is a close kin to hope but it goes a step farther. You must believe in your "heart of hearts", subconscious mind or whatever you call it, that you can get well. You must believe that you can overcome all inhuman terrorists.

4. Faith is a combination of hope and belief amplified to the point it becomes personal power or the ability to take action. When you are sick and under attack by inhuman terrorists it is not easy to fight. It is faith that gives you the ability to do what is necessary to get well. Faith helps you take Transfer Factor and other supplements, get necessary rest, exercise, and get necessary counsel.

5. You must be persistent. Supplements, exercise, and therapy seldom work for people who are not consistent. It requires persistence, day after day, week after week, and year after year, as necessary.

6. You must thirst for and embrace new ideas. You must always be looking for new ideas and accepting of change. I wrote a book called *Herbal Knowledge* a few years ago. At the time, most of the experts agreed with everything in the book. Soy was universally considered a good thing. Today, soy is getting a lot of bad press. Herbal Knowledge states that if you want to lose weight cut out all fat. Many experts still agree, but a growing number say 30% of your calories should come from fat if you want to drop pounds. My book is still considered one of the best, but science has proven that our view of some things has changed and will continue to change.

7. Take personal responsibility. We live in a "blame the other guy" world. "I am miserable because my mother and father got divorced when I was two years old." People tend to blame other people for their own problems. Good or bad, our life is the way it is, either because of what we are doing, what we have done, or who we are. We cannot blame a care-giver because they made a suggestion and we followed it. It is up to us to get the facts, make our own decision, and take action. Only then can we defeat the inhuman terrorists.

Two ways to look at things.
Art Berg was a young man who had everything going for him. His parents were supportive and had the means to give him every material thing he really needed. He was engaged to a beautiful, charming, intelligent, caring woman. Art appeared to have everything a young man could want. But things can change in an instant.

To the world, Art's life appeared to be ruined when the car he was a passenger in crashed. His neck was broken and he was paralyzed from the neck down. He did get some limited use of his arms. Most people would have given up and lived life as a cripple. Not Art, he had an attitude that believed, "It does not matter what happens to you. It matters how you respond to what happens to you."

Art looked at his blessings and what he could do. He did not worry about those things he could not do. He became a public speaker and traveled the world helping people improve their attitude and increase their production. He was remarkably happy and improved the life of almost everyone he touched. When he unexpectedly died of a drug interaction, people came from all over the world to attend his funeral. In a special tribute to Art, they read some of the many words of wisdom he left behind. In a speech, he stated that breaking his neck and changing his life was the best thing that had ever happened to him. He believed he would have gone through life never really making a difference. He died knowing he had made the world a better place. He had more real friends than most people have acquaintances.

Sara Gripealot (name changed to protect the guilty) was a beautiful woman. She had a high IQ, wealthy parents, and tuition paid to any school she wanted to attend. But Sara was not happy. She thought her parents were thoughtless because they insisted she work or go to school. It was unfair of the college to expect her to do the same schoolwork that was expected of students that came from normal families. Her parents were rich so she expected special treatment. When she was convicted for driving under the influence, it was her father's attorney who was at fault. She reasoned that if he had done a better job she would have gotten off.

She died of an intentional overdose of heroin. Her suicide note said, "This world has never been fair. It seems like I have to work to get anything. No one likes me and everyone treats me like I am a burden. I hope you realize that you made me do this. – Sara" Only her family and a dozen or so friends attended her funeral.

The biggest difference between Sara and Art was attitude. Sara was given more. She did not appreciate anything and blamed everyone for her problems. Art looked at everything as a stepping-stone to greater achievement. It is all attitude.

Studies have shown that people with a "poor me" attitude are much more likely to die of cancer or suffer depression. To avoid these two inhuman terrorists, have a great attitude.

Chapter 23
The Never Ending War

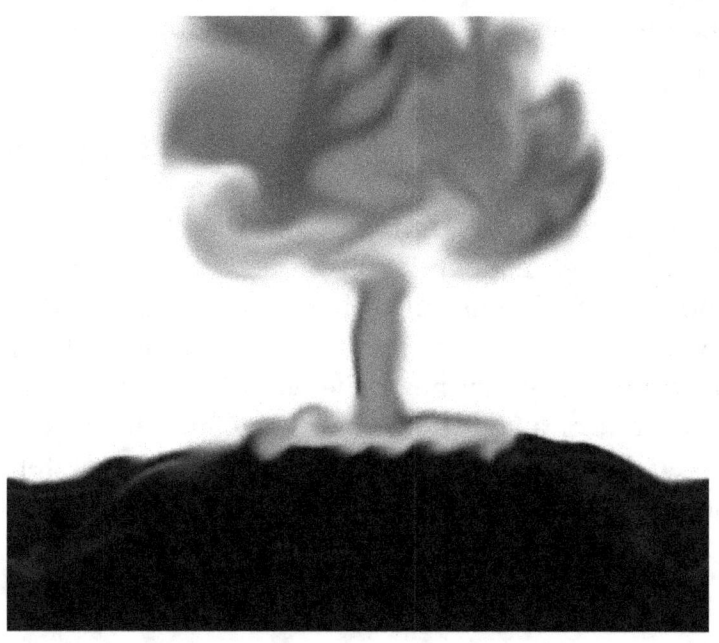

If our species is to survive, the war against inhuman terrorists must be never ending. It is the nature of bacteria, viruses, molds, fungi, and parasites to mutate. As fast as new drugs and inoculations are developed new inhuman terrorists evolve.

Some new terrorists come as a result of drugs and inoculations. Others are developed on purpose by agencies of various world governments. Some governments do it for protection and world peace. Human terrorists rule some countries. These people develop new inhuman terrorists for the sole purpose of instilling fear. As we face the endless onslaught of inhuman terrorists, we must constantly adapt or we will die.

Transfer Factor will educate and strengthen your immune system, but it cannot win the war for you. You are the general who commands and directs your body and your battle. You and you alone control how you respond to outside stimuli. When your spouse cuddles up to you in the middle of the night, you decide whether it makes you angry that he or she would so thoughtlessly wake you out of a sound sleep or makes you feel secure and loved. The first choice will cause you to be agitated and struggle for peace and sleep. The second choice lets you feel safe and sleep well. You are the master.

You are also the quartermaster. You requisition the food, the exercise, the supplements, entertainment, and the junk. In your position as the drill sergeant, you control your learning and your habits. Your habits make you who you are, good or bad. Only you can change them. A phrase I hate to hear as an excuse for bad habits is, "That's just the way I am." You are the way you chose to be. You are the master.

Let Transfer Factor plus its allies help you win every battle. Be aware that God is always there. Use Bee Pollen, Multi Vitamins, and all other tools that aid in your quest for good health, happiness, and long life. Feel good as you eliminate and destroy each and every inhuman terrorist. Most importantly, remember, you are the master!

Glossary of Terms

As used in this book.

Ally or Allies = Any herb, supplement or combination of herbs and supplements that aid the body in healing and enhance the performance of Transfer Factor.

FBI = Health care providers

Inhuman Terrorists = Any harmful virus, bacteria, fungus, mold, parasite, or condition.

Local and State Police = Elements of the immune system. (T-Cells, NK Cells, Macrophages, etc.)

Targeted Transfer Factor = Transfer Factors that target specific conditions.

Transfer factors = Elements found in white blood cells , egg yolks, and colostrum that pass on immunity by educating the immune system.

Transfer Factor = A massive collection of individual transfer factors.

Transfer Factor Plus Allies = Transfer Factor enhanced by Agaricus Blazeii, Beta-Glucan from Baker's Yeast, Beta-Glucan from Oats, Cordyceps sinensis, IP-6 (Inositol hexaphosphate), Maitake Mushroom extract, Mannans (from Aloe Vera leaf), Olive Leaf Extract, Shiitake Mushroom, Soya Bean Extract, and Zinc.

Villain = One of many inhuman terrorists.

References

2003 PDR for Nonprescription Drugs and Dietary Supplements.

"A beta-linked mannan inhibits adherence of Pseudomonas aeruginosa to human lung epithelial cells;" Azghani, A.O.; Williams, I.; Holiday, D.B.; Johnson, A.R.; Glycobiology (1995) 5(1), 39-44.

"A brief review of the immune system;" Alam, R., Prim Care (1998 Dec) 25: 4, 727-38.

"Acemannan, a beta-(1-4)-acctylated mannan, induces nitric oxide production in macrophage cell line RAW 264.7;" Ramamoorthy, J.; Kemp, M.C.; Tizard, J.R.; Mol Pharmacol (1996), 50(4), 878-84.

"A comparison of antibody responses to veterinary vaccine antigens potentiated by different adjuvants;" Usinger, W.R.; Vaccine (1997) 15(17-18), 1902-7.

"A controlled trial of bovine dialyzable leukocyte extract for cryptosporidiosis in patients with AIDS;" McMeeking, A., et al, Journal of Infectious Diseases (1990)

"Acquired wisdom in innate immunity;" Colaco, C., Immunol Today (1998 Jan) 19: 1, 50.

"Active immunization against cancer cells: impediments and advances;" Velders, M.P.; Schreiber, H.; Kast, W.M.; Semin Oncol (1998) 25:6, 697-706.

"Activities and characteristics of transfer factors;" Kirkpatrick, C.H., Biotherapy (1996) 1-3: 13-6.

"Activity of animal transfer factor in man;" Boucheix, Cl et al, Lancet (1977) 198-199.

"Adjuvant treatment using transfer factor for bronchogenic carcinoma: long-term follow-up;" Whyte, R.I., et al, Annals of Thoracic Surgery (1992) 53 (3): 391-6.

"Affect, cognition, the immune system and health;" Kemeny, M.E. and Gruenewald, T.L., Progressive Brain Research (2000) 122: 291-308.

"Aids and Transfer Factor: Myths, Certainties and Realities;" Viza, D.; Biotherapy (1996), 9(1-3), 17-26.

"An ancient system of host defense;" Medzhitov, R., Janeway, C.A., Jr., Curr Opin Immunol (1998) 10: 1, 12-5.

"An In Vitro Screening Study of 196 Natural Products for Toxicity and Efficacy;" See, D.; Gurnee, K.; LeClair, M.; J Am Nutraceutical Assoc (1999) 2(1), 25-41.

"Antibiotic resistance: an ecological imbalance;" Levy, S.B., Ciba Found Symp (1997) 207 (1-9), 1-9;

Antibody Therapy; Wawrzynczak, E.J.; Oxford, UK: BIOS Scientific Publishers Limited (1995) p. 9-10.

"Antitumor activity exhibited by orally administered extract from fruit body of Grifola frondosa (maitake);" Hishida, I; Nanba, H.; Kuroda, H.; Chem Pharm Bull (Tokyo) (1988) 36:5, 1819-27.

"Antitumor activity of orally administered 'D-fraction' from maitake mushroom (Grifola frondosa);" Nanba, H., Journal of Naturopathic Medicine (1993) 4: 10-15.

"Antitumor mechanisms of orally administered shitake fruit bodies;" Nanba, H.; Kuroda, H.; Chem Pharm Bull (Tokyo) (1987) 35(6), 2459-64.

"Augmentation of various immune reactivities of tumor-bearing hosts with an extract of Cordyceps sinensis;" Yamaguchi, N.; Yoshida, J.; Ren, L.J.; Chen, H.; Miyazawa, Y.; Fujii, Y.; Huang, Y.X.; Takamura, S.; Suzuki, S.; Koshimura, S.; et al Biotherapy (1990)

"Autoaggression and tumor rejection: it takes more than self-specific T-cell activation;" Ganss, R.; Limmer, A.; Sacher, T.; Arnold, B.; Hemmerling, G.J.; Immunol Rev (1999) 169, 263-72.

"Biological response modifiers. Interferons, interleukins, and transfer factor;" Kirkpatrick, C.H., Annals of Allergy (1989) 62(3): 170-6.

"Breastfeeding Stimulates the Infant Immune System;" Hanson, L.A.; Science and Medicine (1997) 2-11.

"Clinical Study of P-TFOL Liquid Treating Hepatitis;" Wu Jing Xing; Jiang Jia Kun; XIth International Congress on Transfer Factor, (1-4 Mar 1999) Monterrey, MX.

"Comparison of pure inositol hexaphosphate and high-bran diet in the prevention of DMBA-induced rat mammary carcinogensis;" Vuccenik, J.; Yang, G.Y.; Shamsuddin, A.M.; Nutr Cancer (1997) 28:1, 7-13.

"Complement and its role in immune response;" Hess, C., Steiger, J.U., Schifferli, J.A., Schweiz Med Wochenschr (1998) 128: 11, 393-9.

"Complement factors and their receptors;" Ember, J. A., Hugli, T.E., Immunopharmacology (1997), 38, 3-15.

"Complement and immunity to viruses;" Lachmann, P. J., Davies, A., Immunological Reviews (1997),

"Cytokine and Lymphocyte Levels in Extrinsic Asthma Patients Treated with Transfer Factor;" Enciso, J.A.; Miranda, F.S.; Gomez-Martinez, J.C.; Portuguez-Diaz, A.; Badillo, A.; Orea-S, M.; Gomez-Vera, J.; Flores-Sandoval, G.; Estrada-Patra, S.; XIth International Congress on Transfer Factor, (1-4 Mar 1999) Monterrey, MX.

"Double-blind placebo-controlled pilot trial of accmannan in advanced human immunodeficiency virus disease;" Montaner, J.S.; Gill, J.; Singer, J.; Kaboud, J.; Arseneau, R.; McLean, B.D.; Schechter, M.T.; Ruedy, J.; J Acquir Immune Defic Syndr Hum Retrovirol (1996) 12(2), 153-7.

"Effect of in vitro produced transfer factor on the immune response of cancer patients;" Pizza, G., et al, European Journal of Cancer (1977) 13, 917-923.

"Effect of Jinshuibao capsule on the immunological function of 36 patients with advanced cancer;" Zhou, D.H.; Lin, L.Z.; Chung Kuo Chung, I.; Isi, I.; Chieh Ho Tsa Chih (1995) 15:8, 476-8.

"Efficacy of the Transfer Factor in the Severely Infected Pediatric Patient;" Ayala-de la Cruz, M.C.; Rodriguez-Padilla, C.; Tamez-Guerra, R.; XIth International Congress on Transfer Factor, (1-4 Mar 1999) Monterrey, MX.

Enhanced Transfer Factor. William J. Hennen Ph.D., Woodland Publishing.

"Eleventh International Congress on Transfer Factors;" Dumonde DC, et al, March 1-4, 1999, Monterrey, Nuevo Leon, Mexico Journal of Interferon Cytokine Research (2000 April) 20(4): 439-41.

"Evasion of pathogens by avoiding recognition or eradication by complement, in part via molecular mimicry;" Wurzner, R.; Mol Immunol (1999), 36: 4-5, 249-60.

"Evidence that stress and surgical interventions promote tumor development by suppressing Natural Killer cell activity;" Ben Eliyahu, S.; Page, G.G.; Yirmiya, R.; Shakhar, G.; Int J. Cancer (1999) 80: 6, 880-8.

"Experience with Transfer Factor with 60 Patients in ICU;" Sergio, G.G.; XIth International Congress on Transfer Factor, (1-4 Mar 1999) Monterrey, MX.

"Functional properties of edible mushrooms;" Chang, R.; Nutr Rev (1996) 54 (11 Pr 2), 591-3.

"Human Natural Killer cells;" Barpo, I, Ascenspo, J.L., Arch Immunol Ther Exp (Warsz) (1998) 46:4, 213-29.

"Human Natural Killer cells in health and disease;" Biology and therapeutic potential, Whiteside, T.L., Herberman, R.B., Clin Immunother (1994), 1: 1, 56-66.

"Immune-enhancing agent for therapeutic use in immunocompromised hosts;" Beardsley, T.R.; USP 5,616,554 (1 Apr 1997).

Immunology, Eighth Ed., Weir, D.M.; Stewart, J.; Churchill Livingstone, New York (1997), p. 261.

Immunology, Fourth Ed., Riott I., Brostoff J., Male D., Mosby, London (1996).

"Immunoregulartory Activities of Oat b-Glucan In vitro and In vivo;" Estrada, A.; Yn, C-H.; Van Kessel, A.; Li, B.; Hauta, S.; Laarveld, B.; Microbial Immunol (1997)

"Increased adiposity in animals due to a human virus;" Dhurandhar, NV. International Journal of Obesity and Related Metabolic Disorders, (2000 Aug.)

"Infections, atherosclerosis, and coronary heart disease;" Famularo, G., Annals of the Italian Medical Institute (2000 Apr-Jun) 15(2): 144-55.

"Influence of oral zinc supplementation on the lymphocyte response to mitogens of normal subjects;" Duchateau J., et al, American Journal of Clinical Nutrition (1981)

"Inositol hexaphosphate inhibits growth and induces differentiation of PC-3 human prostate cancer cells;" Shamsuddia, A.M.; Yang, G.Y.; Carcinogenesis (1995) 16:8, 1975-9.

"Inositol phosphates have novel anticancer function;" Shamsuddia, A.M.; J Nutr (1995)

"Insect immunity: evolutionary roots of the mammalian innate immune system;" Vilmos, P., Kurucz, F., Immunol Lett (1998) 62: 2, 59-66.

"In vitro studies during long-term oral administration of specific Transfer Factor;" Pizza, G.; De Vinci, C.; Fornarola, V.; Palareti, A.; Baricordi, O.; Viza, D.; Biotherapy (1996) 9 (1-3), 175-85.

"IP6: a novel anti-cancer agent;" Shamsuddin, A.M.; Vucenik, I.; Cole, K.E.; Life Sci (1997) 61:4, 343-54.

"IP6-induced growth inhibition and differentiation of HT-29 human colon cancer cells: involvement of intracellular inositol phosphates;" Yang, G.Y.; Shamsuddia, A.M.; Anticancer Res (1995) 15:6B, 2479-87.

"IP6 in treatment of liver cancer. II. Intra-tumoral injection of IP6 regresses pre-existing human liver cancer xenotransplanted in nude mice;" Vucenik, I.; Zhang, Z.S.; Shamsuddin, A.M.; Anticancer Res (1998)

"Linkages of innate and adaptive immunity;" Carroll, M.C.; Prodeus, A. P.; Curr Opin Immunol (1998)

"Long-term remission of malignant brain tumors after intracranial infection: a report of four cases;" Bowles, A.P., Jr.; Perkins, E.; Neurosurgery (1999 Mar) 44:3, 636-42; discussion 642-3.

"Management of Hypercosinophilia with the Transfer Factor;" Ayala-de la Cruz, M.C.; Rodriguez-Padilla, C.; Tamez-Guerra, R.; XIth International Congress on Transfer Factor, (1-4 Mar 1999) Monterrey, MX.

"Medicinal and therapeutic value of the shitake mushroom;" Jong, S.C.; Birmingham, J.M.; Adv Appl Microbiol (1993) 39, 153-84.

"Medicinal fungi of the world;" Pengelly, A., Modern Phytotherapist (1996) 2: 1, 3-8.

"Murine Transfer Factors: dose-response relationships and routes of administration;" Kirkpatrick, C.H.; Harnad, A.R.; Morton, I.C.; Cell Immunol (1995) 164(2)

"Natural Killer cells and Natural Killer cell activity in chronic fatigue syndrome;" Whiteside, T.L.; Friberg D. Am J. Med (1998) 105: 3A, 27S-34S.

"Observation of 26 Senile Cases Treated with P-TFOL;" Wang
Huifang; Zhou Guanghua; Yu Zhiying; Xu Yonggang; Jiang
Jia Kun; XIth International Congress on Transfer Factor, (1-4
Mar 1999) Monterrey, MX.
"Observation of the effect of PSTF oral liquor on the positive
tuberculin test reaction;" Wu S.; Zhong X.; Chung Kuo, I.;
Hsuch Ko, I.; Isueh Yan Hsueh Pao (1992)
"Oral bovine Transfer Factor (OTF) use in the hyper-IgE syndrome;"
Jones, J.F.; et al. In: Immunobiology of Transfer Factor;
Academic Press; New York (1983)
"Orally administered specific transfer factor for the treatment of
herpes infections;" Viza, D., et al, Lymphok Res (1985) 4, 27-
30.
"Peptide Sequences That Are Common to Transfer Factors;"
Kirkpatrick, C.H.; XIth International Congress on Transfer
Factor, (1-4 Mar 1999) Monterrey, MX.
"Pilot study of the effect of acemannan in cats infected with feline
immunodeficiency virus;" Yates, K.M.; Rosenberg, I.J.;
Harris, C.K.; Bronstad, D.C.; King, G.K.; Biehle, G.A.;
Walker, B.; For, C.R.; Hall, J.F.; Tizard, I.R.; Vet-Immunol-
Immunopathol (1992) 35(1-2), 177-89.
"Potentiation of host-mediated antitumor activity in mice by beta-
glucan obtained from Grifola frondosa (maitake);" Adachi,
K.; Nanba, H.; Kuroda, H.; Chem Pharm Bull (Tokyo) (1987)
35(1), 262-70.
"Process for obtaining transfer factor from colostrums transfer factor
so obtained and use thereof;" Wilson, G.B.; Paddock, G.V.;
US Patent Number 4816563
"Randomized controlled trial of transfer factor
immunochemotherapy as an adjunct to surgical treatment
for primary adenocarcinoma of the lung;" Fujisawa, T.,
et al, Japanese Journal of Surgery (1984)
"Reasons for the emergence of antibiotic resistence;" Tenover, F.C.,
McGowan, J.F., Jr., Am J Med Sci (1996)
"Reduction in virus-neutralizing activity of a bovine colostrums
immunoglobulin concentrate by gastric acid and digestive
enzymes;" Petschow, B.W.; Talbott, R.D.; J Pediatr
Gastroenterol Nutr (1994) 19, 228-35.

"Reduction of cell proliferation and enhancement of NK-cell activity;" Shamsuddia, A.M.; United States Patent 5,082,833; Jan 21, 1992.

"Regulatory mechanisms of NK cell functions;" Toyama, Sorimachi N., Koyasu, S., Nippon Rinsho (1999)

"Regulatory T cells in thymic epithelium-induced tolerance. I. Suppression of mature peripheral non-tolerant T cells;" Modigliani, Y.; Pereira, P.; Thomas, Vaslin V.; Salan, J.; Burlen, Defranoux, O.; Coutinho, A.; Le Douarin, N.; Bandeira, A.; Fur J Immunol (1995) 25:9, 2563-71.

"Return to the past: the case for antibody-based therapies in infectious diseases;" Casadevall, A., Scharff, M.D.; Clinical Infections Diseases (1995) 21, 150-61.

"Review of the evidence for an association between infant feeding and childhood cancer;" Davis, M.K.; Int J Cancer Suppl (1998) 11: 29-33.

"Role of human Natural Killer cells in health and disease;" Whiteside, T.L.; Herberman, R. B.; Clin Diagn Lab Immunol (1994) 1: 2, 125-33.

"Role of Natural Killer cells in innate resistance to protozoan infections;" Scharton Kersten, T.M.; Sher, A.; Curr Opin Immunol (1997) 9: 1, 44-51.

"Shaking up immunity: psychological and immunologic changes after a natural disaster;" [see comments] Solomon, G.F.; Segerstrom, S.C.; Grohr, P.; Kemeny, M.; Fahey, J.; Psychosom Med. (1997) 59: 2, 114-27.

"Specific transfer factor protects mice against lethal challenge with herpes simplex virus;" Viza, D., et al, Cellular Immunity (1986) 100, 555-562.

"Specific transfer factor with activity against Epstein-Barr virus reduces late relapse in endemic Burkitt's lymphoma;" Neequaye, J., et al, Anticancer Research (1990) 10(5A): 1183-7.

"Structural nature and functions of transfer factors." Kirkpatrick, C.H., Ann N Y Acad. Sci., (1993 Jun 23)

"Successful Treatment of Neuritis Posherperca (Caused by Herpes Zoster) with Specific Transfer Factor;" Ondarza, R.; Chavez, R.; Serrano, E.; Correa, B.; Ramirez, R.; Estrada-G, I.; Estrada-Parra, S.; XIth International Congress on Transfer Factor, (1-4 Mar 1999) Monterrey, MX.

"Suppression of Natural Killer cell activity in patients with fracture/soft tissue injury;" Hauser, C.J.; Joshi, P.; Jones, Q.; Zhou, X.; Livingston, D.H.; Lavery, R.F.; Arch Surg (1997) 132: 12, 1326-30.

"Suppurative Adenopathy by Salmonell B Treated with Transfer Factor. Case Report;" Berron, R.; Almendarez, C.; Rosiles, G.; XIth International Congress on Transfer Factor, (1-4 Mar 1999) Monterrey, MX.

"Targeting of Natural Killer cells to mammary carcinoma via naturally occurring tumor cell-bound iC3b and beta-glucan primed CR3 (CD11b/CD18);" Vetvicka, V.; Thornton, B.P.; Wieman, T.J.; Ross, G.D.; J Immunol (1997) 159:2, 599-605.

"TF, Psoriasis and Cytokines;" Wang yuying; Liu Zhenxiang; Shen Li; XIth International Congress on Transfer Factor, (1-4 Mar 1999) Monterrey, MX.

"The absorption of colostral immunoglobulins in newborn piglets. II Effect of water or glucose solutions on the permeability of the newborn intestine;" Klobasa, F.; Habe, F.; Wehahn, E.; Berl Munch Tierarztl Wochenschr (1991) 104, 37-41.

"The adjuvant and specific activity of transfer factors to Candida albicans;" Borysov VA et al Fiziol Z (1998)

"The adjuvant therapy of nasopharyngeal tumor with transfer factor;" Sibl, O., et al, Research and Application of Transfer Factor and DLE (1989) 403-10.

"The beta-glucan binding lectin site of mouse CR3 (CD11b/CD18) and its function in generating a primed state of the receptor that mediates cytotoxic activation in response to iC3b-opsonized targe cells;" Xia, Y.; Vetvicka, V.; Yan, J.; Hanikyrova, M.; Mayadas, T.N.; Ross, G.D.; J Immunol (1999) 162:4, 2281-90.

"The cellular transfer of cutaneous Hypersensitivity to tuberculin in man;" Lawrence, H.S.; Proc Soc Exp Biol Med (1949) 71, 516.

"The clinical uses of specific transfer factors;" Pekarek, J., et al, Recent Advances in Transfer factors and Dailyzable Leukocyte Extracts (1992) 256-63.

"The cost of not breastfeeding: a commentary;" Riodan, J.M.; J Hum Lact (1997) 13(2), 93-7.

"The effects of yeast polysaccharides on mouse tumors;" Diller, I.C.; Mankowski, Z.T., Fisher, M.E.; Cancer Res (1963) 23:201.

"The role of Natural Killer cells in viral infections;" see DM; Khemka, P.; Sahl, I.; Bui, T.; Tilles, J.G.; Scand J Immunol (1997) 46: 3, 217-24.

"The scientific rediscovery of an ancient Chinese herbal medicine: Cordyceps sinensis: part I;" Zhu, J.S.; Halpern, G.M.; Jones, K.; J Altern Complement Med (1998) 4(3), 289-303.

"The scientific rediscovery of a precious ancient Chinese herbal medicine: Cordyceps sinensis: part II;" Zhu, J.S.; Halpern, G.M.; Jones, K.; J Altern Complement Med (1998) 4(4), 429-457.

"The Transfer Factor in the Management of a Case of Encephalitis Caused by Coccidioides Immitis;" Ayala-de la Cruz, M.C.; Rodriguez-Padilla, C.; Tamez-Guerra, R.; XIth International Congress on Transfer Factor, (1-4 Mar 1999) Monterrey, MX.

"The Use of Transfer Factor in a Case of Refractive Urinary Tract Infection;" Ayala-de la Cruz, M.C.; Rodriguez-Padilla, C.; Tamez-Guerra, R.; XIth International Congress on Transfer Factor, (1-4 Mar 1999) Monterrey, MX.

"The use of transfer factors in the treatment of multiple sclerosis: a case report;" Sacks, N., et al, South Africa Medical Journal (1976 Sep 18) 50 (40): 1556-8.

"Therapeutic effects of substances occurring in higher Basidiomycetes mushrooms: a modern perspective;" Wasser, S.P.; Weis, A.L.; Crit Rev Immunol (1999)

"Therapeutic intervention with complement and beta-glucan in cancer;" Ross, G.D.; Vetvicka, V.; Yan, J.; Xia, Y.; Vitvickova, J.; Immunopharmacology (1999) 42:1-3, 61-74.

"Therapeutic potential of transfer factor;" Kirkpatrick, C.H., [editorial], New England Journal of Medicine (1980) 14; 303(7): 390-1.

"Thymus function, ageing and autoimmunity;" Rose, N.R.; Immunol Lett (1994) 40(3), 225-30.

"Transfer factor 1993: New frontiers;" Fudenberg, H.H.; Pizza, G.; Progress in Drug Res (1994) 42, 309-400.

"Transfer Factor current status and future prospects;" Lawrence, H.S.; Borkowsky, W.; Biotherapy (1996) 9(1-3), 1-5.

Transfer Factor; Hennen, William J., Woodland, Pleasant Grove, Utah, 1998.

"Transfer Factor and its clinical application;" Schulkind, M.L. and Ayoub, E.M., Advanced Pediatrics (1980) 27: 89-115.

"Transfer factor as an adjuvant to non-small cell lung cancer;" Pilotti, V., et al, Biotherapy, (1996) 9 (1-3): 117-121.

"Transfer Factor as a Good Therapeutic Agent in Moderate and Severe Atopic Dermatitis;" Navarro-Cruz, D.; Serrano-Miranda, E.; Orea-S, M.; Estrada-Parra, S.; Teran-Ortiz, I.; Gomez-Vera, J.; Flores-Sandoval, G.; XIth International Congress on Transfer Factor, (1-4 Mar 1999) Monterrey, MX.

"Transfer factor for the prevention of varicella-zoster infection in childhood leukemia;" Steele, R.W., et al, New England Journal of Medicine (1980) 14; 303(7): 355-9.

"Transfer factor for the treatment of HbsAg-positive chronic active hepatitis. P. Soc. Exp. Med. (1985) 178, 468-475.

"Transfer Factor (Immodin Seva) Treatment of Recurrent Anterior Uveitis B a Retrospective Evaluation after Ten Years;" Hana, I.; Star, J.; Boguszakova, J.; Pekarek, J.; Ivaskova, E.; XIth International Congress on Transfer Factor, (1-4 Mar 1999) Monterrey, MX.

"Transfer factor in Malignancy;" Pizza, G.; De Vinci, C.; Fudengerg, H.H.; Progress in Drug Res (1994), 42, 401-421.

"Transfer Factor in the Era of AIDS;" Pizza, G.; Viza D.; Biotherapy (1996) 9 (1-3), ix-x.

"Transfer Factor: Past, Present and Future;" Fudengerg, H.H.; Ann Rev Pharm Tox (1989) 475-516.

Transfer Factor Institute web site, Richard Bennett, Ph.D.

Transfer Factors. Rita Elkins M.H., Woodland Publishing.

"Transfer factors: identification of conserved sequences in transfer factor molecules;" Kirkpatrick, C.H., Molecular Medicine (2000 April) 6(4): 332-41.

"Treatment of Atopic Dermatitis with Transfer Factor and Cyclosporin A.;" Cordero-Miranda, M.A.; Serrano-Miranda, E.; Flores-Sandoval, G.; Gomez-Vera, J.; Orea-S, M.; Correa-Meaz, B.; Ramirez, R.; Badillow-Flores, A.; Estrada-Parra, S.; XIth International Congress on Transfer Factor, (1-4 Mar 1999) Monterrey, MX.

"Treatment of diarrhea in human immunodeficiency virus-infected patients with immunoglobulins from bovine colostrums;" Rump, J.A.; Arndt, R.; Arnold, A.; Bendick, C.; Dichtelmuller, H.; Franke, M.; Helm, F.B.; Jager, H.; Kampmann, B.; Kolb, P.; et al; Clin Investig (1992) 70, 588-94.

"Treatment of Mycobacterium-fortuitum pulmonary infection with
    Transfer Factor: New methodology for evaluating TF
    potency and predicting clinical response;" Wilson, G.B., et al,
    Clinical Immunology and Immunopathology (1982) 23: 478.
"Twenty-five Years of Clinical Experience with Transfer Factor;"
    Pizza, G.; De Vinci, C.; Palareti, A.; Viza, D.;
    XIth International Congress on Transfer Factor, (1-4 Mar
    1999) Monterrey, MX.
carcinoma cell line;" Saied, I.T.; Shamsuddia, A.M.; Anticancer Res
    (1998) 18:3A, 1479-84.

Notes:

_____

_____

_____

_____

_____

_____

_____

_____

_____

_____

Other Books by Clive Buchanan:

18 Steps to Greatness
One Man's Victory, Multiple Sclerosis
Herbal Knowledge
Walking with Lions
Love, Money, and Personal Power

To book Clive Buchanan as a speaker
call: 1-435-275-6649 or 1-888-344-3892
Website: ask4clive.com
E-mail: clive@ask4clive.com